Dash Diet Cookbook for Beginners:

555 Amazing and Simple Recipes for 2020. Lose Weight Fast, Easy and in Healthy Way!

Table Of Contents

Introduction..5

Chapter 1 – All about the DASH Eating Plan..7

Chapter 2 – Appetizer Recipes.............53

Chapter 3 – Breakfast Recipes..............72

Chapter 4 – Main Course Recipes........93

Chapter 5 – Salad Recipes...................108

Chapter 6 – Dessert and Beverage Recipes...124

Chapter 7 – Recipes for Snacks and Side Dish...173

Chapter 8 – Soup Recipes...................225

Conclusion...265

© Copyright July Anderson 2019 - All rights reserved.

The content contained within this book may not be reproduced, duplicated or transmitted without direct written permission from the author or the publisher.

Under no circumstances will any blame or legal responsibility be held against the publisher, or author, for any damages, reparation, or monetary loss due to the information contained within this book, either directly or indirectly.

Legal Notice:

This book is copyright protected. It is only for personal use. You cannot amend, distribute, sell, use, quote or paraphrase any part, or the content within this book, without the consent of the author or publisher.

Disclaimer Notice:

Please note the information contained within this document is for educational and entertainment purposes only. All effort has been executed to present accurate, up to date, reliable, complete information. No warranties of any kind are declared or implied. Readers acknowledge that the author is not engaging in the rendering of legal, financial, medical or professional advice. The content within this book has been derived from various sources. Please consult a licensed professional before attempting any techniques outlined in this book.

By reading this document, the reader agrees that under no circumstances is the author responsible for any losses, direct or indirect, that are incurred as a result of the use of information contained within this document, including, but not limited to, errors, omissions, or inaccuracies.

Introduction

This book contains all you need to know about the DASH eating plan – its benefits, how to start, and delectable recipes that will inspire you to commit to the plan.

DASH stands for Dietary Approaches to Stop Hypertension. It is more of a lifestyle than a diet. This eating plan teaches you what to eat to sustain your body with the right amounts of nutrients. It keeps you focused on making sure that you don't get too much calories and sodium – two factors that affect blood pressure and heart health.

This eating plan has lots of health benefits and unlike fad diets, this will not make you feel deprived. You only have to make adjustments to what you are eating, especially if you aren't used to eating fruits and vegetables. This book has 555 recipes that you can try to help you on your journey towards a healthier and fitter version of yourself. This book also offers important information about the DASH eating plan and a 7-day sample eating plan.

Thanks for downloading this book, I hope you enjoy it!

Chapter 1 – All about the DASH Eating Plan

According to research, one out of 3 adults in the US suffers from high blood pressure. About 59 million or 28 percent of the country's population experience prehypertension, a medical condition that can lead to stroke and heart ailment.

High blood pressure is a condition when the blood pressure stays elevated longer than usual. It is usually caused by your weight, foods you eat, sodium intake, improper stress management, smoking, alcohol consumption and level of your physical activity.

You have to make two vital changes in your diet to maintain a healthy level of blood pressure. First, you have to eat less sodium or salt and you need to follow the DASH eating plan.

DASH stands for Dietary Approaches to Stop Hypertension. It is an eating plan that aims to maintain healthy levels of blood pressure by being mindful of your calorie and sodium intake.

This eating plan includes nuts, poultry, fish, whole grains, fruits, veggies, and low-fat milk. Here are the other important rules in this kind of an eating plan:

- Eat veggies rich in protein like cooked legumes, such as chickpeas, lentils, and kidney beans.
- It is rich in calcium, potassium, magnesium and high in fiber.
- Reduce your intake of sweetened drinks, sweets, and red meat.
- Limit your intake of sodium or salt to 2000mg per day.
- You'll consume foods with low content of cholesterol, saturated fat, and total fat.

The Benefits of the Diet

Through several studies and trials, researchers conclude that the DASH eating plan offers the following health benefits:

1. Lower blood pressure. Expect a few points drop in your blood pressure within a couple of weeks after starting with the diet. Expect more points to drop in your systolic blood pressure after a month or two. If you will make this eating plan a part of your lifestyle, you will experience its long-term effect – maintaining a healthy level of blood pressure.

2. Reduce your risk of cancer. This is because the diet requires you to eat a lot of fresh or frozen vegetables and fruits.

3. Stronger bones. Aside from improving bone strength, you'll also have a lower risk of suffering from osteoporosis. This is due to the high amounts of calcium you get from green leafy vegetables and dairy products.

4. Lower risk of suffering from gout. The eating plan reduces a person's uric acid levels.

5. Decrease in the LDL and total cholesterol in the blood. As a result, you will have regular blood pressure and you'll also have a lower risk of suffering from cerebrovascular disease and metabolic disorders, including diabetes and cardiovascular disease.

This is not a deprivation diet. If you want to lose weight as you follow the eating plan, you have to be mindful of the portions of your meals. You must also make it a habit to exercise.

Getting Started

You need to commit to a lot of changes in your diet, especially if you are used to eating too much salty, fatty, and junk foods. Once you have set your mind in following the DASH diet plan, you can gradually commit to the changes. Start with one or two of the following dietary changes until your system has gotten used to the plan:

- If you aren't fond of vegetables, make an effort to add an extra serving of veggies on your every meal.
- To make it easier for you to remember adding veggies to your dishes, you can prepare them ahead of time. Wash and cut them before putting in a clean container. Place in the fridge until ready to use. You can easily put the prepared veggies on sauces, soups, stir-fried dishes or casseroles.
- Try to consume more grains, veggies, and legumes than meat. You can try tweaking meat recipes by adding more of these ingredients than meat.
- Whole grain products are rich in fiber. Choose this kind whenever necessary because whole grains can make you feel full at a faster rate.
- In filling your plate, make sure that you have larger portions of whole grain products and vegetables than fish, poultry or meat.
- Stock up on low-fat milk. You can add it to soups and cooked cereals. You can also drink it as a substitute for sweetened drinks. It is also necessary to include this kind of milk with meals.

- Avoid eating processed foods. Do not add more than the required amount of salt when cooking. Keep the salt shaker out of reach when eating so that you won't be tempted to add more to your meals.
- Snack on fresh and dried fruits, a small piece of low-fat cheese or low-fat yogurt.

If you aren't used to eating too much fiber, make sure that you slowly add foods rich in fiber to your diet. You must also increase your water intake up to 10 cups per day as you increase your fiber intake. Too much fiber in the diet without supplying your system with enough fluids may result in constipation, diarrhea, cramping, bloating, and gas.

Vital Lifestyle Changes to Lower Blood Pressure

A person's blood pressure is recorded as two numbers and measured in mm Hg or millimeters of mercury. The number on top is called the systolic blood pressure, which is your blood pressure when your heart is contracting or working. The number on the lower portion is called the diastolic blood pressure. It is the blood pressure measurement when your heart is in a relaxed state.

The normal blood pressure for individuals varies on your health condition, age, and other factors that only your doctor can determine. There is a general guideline though as per the Canadian Hypertension Program Recommendations published in 2015. It states that normal blood pressure levels include the following:

- Less than 50 systolic blood pressure for people 80 years old and above
- Less than 130/80 mm Hg for adults suffering from diabetes
- Less than 140/90 mm Hg for most adults including people suffering from chronic kidney disease

Here are the recommended lifestyle changes you can do and how they can affect your blood pressure:

- Lose weight, if needed. - You'll experience a drop of 1 mm Hg for your systolic and diastolic blood pressure.
- Limit your alcohol consumption to no more than 1 drink per day for women and 2 drinks per day for men. - You'll experience a drop of 4 mm Hg for systolic and 2 mm Hg for diastolic blood pressure.

- Make it a habit to exercise, including an hour of heart-beat rising movements at least 4 times a week. - You'll experience a drop of 5 mm Hg for systolic and 4 mm Hg for diastolic blood pressure.
- Follow the DASH eating plan. - You'll experience a drop of 16 mm Hg for systolic and 8 mm Hg for diastolic blood pressure.

Maintain healthy levels of your blood pressure by reducing stress and quit vices bad for the health, including smoking.

All about Sodium

Sodium is a mineral found in table salt. Most of the sodium many people get comes from fast and processed foods. According to the 1991 published article in the Journal of the American College Nutrition, 77 percent of sodium is added during processing, 12 percent are naturally found in foods and 11 percent come from table salt and added while cooking.

Make it a habit to read the Nutrition Facts usually found at the back of most food packages. It contains the amount of nutrients, including sodium, you'll get in one serving and its percentage Daily Value. The general guideline for sodium to be considered as a small amount when listed in the percentage Daily Value is 5 percent or less.

The healthy levels of sodium coming from both food and drinks recommended each day are 5 percent or less.

Choosing the Right Foods with Less Sodium Content

Here's a list of the foods to eat and stay away from in following the DASH eating plan:

1. Fruits

To eat:

- All fruit juices
- Most fresh, canned or frozen fruits

Limit your intake:

- Certain dried and processed fruits with salt and other ingredients with sodium

2. Vegetable

To eat:

- All kinds of vegetables (fresh and frozen)
- Homemade mashed potatoes

- Salt-free or low sodium vegetable juice
- Low sodium canned veggies
- Homemade pasta sauce
- Canned vegetables (drained)

Limit your intake:

- Pasta sauce (in jar or can)
- Regular tomato or vegetable juice
- Instant mashed potatoes
- Veggies seasoned with salted pork, bacon or ham
- Foods prepared in brine, pickled veggies, pickles, sauerkraut
- Canned vegetable (regular and undrained)

3. Cereals, bread, and grains

To eat:

- Quinoa, barley, rice, millet, kasha, bulgur, couscous
- Homemade or low-sodium breadcrumbs
- Homemade bread stuffing
- Pasta, macaroni, spaghetti
- Unsalted rice cakes, breadsticks, crackers
- Cooked cereals (without added salt)

- Most dry cereals (with 200mg salt per serving or less)
- Homemade cornbread and muffins
- Bread and rolls (whole grains)

Limit your intake:

- Packaged rice and pasta mixes
- Packaged cracker crumbs or breadcrumbs
- Packaged bread stuffing
- Dry cereals (with more than 200mg salt per serving)
- Self-rising flour and biscuit mixes
- Waffles (frozen and mixes)
- Pancakes (frozen and mixes)
- Instant hot cereals
- Packages bread and muffin mixes
- Crackers, rolls, and breads with salted tops

4. Fats

To eat:

- Light cream cheese
- Light cream
- Regular and low-sodium salad dressings
- Light sour cream

- Unsaturated vegetable oils
- Non-hydrogenated margarine

Limit your intake:

- Commercially prepared gravies and sauces
- Snack dips made with processed cheese or instant soup mixes
- Regular salad dressings with salted pork, bacon bits, and bacon fat

5. Soups

To eat:

- Commercially dehydrated and canned broths, bouillons (with less than 500mg sodium per serving)
- Homemade soups and broths (without added salt)

Limit your intake:

- Regular bouillon liquid, powder or cubes, and dry soup mixes
- Regular broths or bouillon and canned soups

6. Meat and alternatives

To eat:

- Most shellfish, fresh or frozen fish, poultry, pork, lamb, and beef
- Canned tuna (drained and rinsed)
- Canned salmon (low sodium)
- Unflavored egg substitutes and eggs
- Unsalted or regular peanut butter
- Dried lentils, beans, and peas
- Unsalted nuts and seeds

Limit your intake:

- Frozen breaded meats
- Pickled, salted, cured or smoked meats - canned meats, luncheon meat, pickled herring, bacon, ham, hotdogs, sausages
- Pickled eggs
- Regular cottage cheese
- Pot pies (store-bought or commercial)
- Canned baked beans
- Salted nuts

7. Milk and alternatives

To eat:

- Ricotta cheese

- Low-fat yogurt
- Light cheese or partly skimmed hard cheese
- Soy milk
- Milk (including eggnog and chocolate milk)

Limit your intake:

- Regular sauces, cheese spreads, and hard, processed cheese
- Milkshake, malted milk, buttermilk

8. Other

To eat:

- Carbonated beverages
- Unsalted popcorn and pretzels
- Low sodium tortilla chips
- Horseradish (fresh ground)
- Lime or lemon juice
- Vinegar
- Spices and herbs
- Pepper
- Salt substitute (with doctor's approval)
- Seasonings (with no salt added)

Limit to 1 serving per day:

- 1 tablespoon of mustard
- 1 tablespoon of ketchup
- 1 tablespoon of relish
- 1 tablespoon of barbecue sauce
- 1 serving (as labeled) low sodium soy sauce
- 1/2 teaspoon reduced-sodium soy sauce
- 2 tablespoon salsa
- 1 teaspoon hot pepper sauce

Limit your intake:

- Monosodium glutamate
- Meat coating mixes
- Meat tenderizers
- Kosher salt
- Rock salt
- Sea salt
- Any seasoning made with salt - lemon pepper, seasoned salt, onion salt, celery salt, garlic salt
- Instant cake and pudding mixes
- Artificial fruit-flavored crystals (with sodium or salt in the ingredients)
- Softened water used for cooking or drinking
- Olives
- salted snack foods
- Canned grave and mixes

- Hoisin sauce
- Black bean sauce
- Worcestershire sauce
- Steak sauce
- Teriyaki sauce
- Regular soy sauce

Being Mindful of Your Calorie Intake

Aside from the health benefits, DASH can also help you achieve your weight goals. You only have to be mindful of your calorie intake. Eat more fruits and vegetables than foods rich in calories, such as sweets.

Here are some samples on how you can keep an eye of your calorie consumption:

1. Increase intake of low-fat or fat-free milk products.

- Instead of consuming half a cup of full-fat ice cream, eat half a cup of low-fat frozen yogurt. This will save you 70 calories.

2. Eat more vegetables.

- Instead of consuming 5 ounces of chicken, eat half a cup of raw veggies with 2 ounces of chicken, stir-fried using

a little amount of vegetable oil. This will save you 50 calories.
- Instead of eating hamburger with 6 ounces of meat, retain half the meat and add half a cup of spinach and half a cup of carrots. This will save you about 200 calories.

3. Eat more fruits.

- Instead of munching on a 2-ounce bag of pork rinds, eat 1/4 cup of dried apricots. This will save you 230 calories.
- Instead of eating 4 shortbread cookies, snack on a medium-sized apple. This will save you 80 calories.

Here are the other tips you can follow to save more calories:

- Drink club soda or water with a wedge of lime or lemon.
- Eat unsalted and unbuttered rice cakes or popcorn, vegetable sticks, and fruits as snacks.
- Limit consumption of foods with too much added sugar, including fruit drinks, regular soft drinks, sherbet, ice

cream, candy bars, flavored yogurts, and pies.
- Eat fruits canned in water or in their own juice.
- You can mix fruits to plain low-fat or fat-free yogurt.
- Make it a habit to compare food labels, especially the nutrition fact content of packaged foods. Not because a food item claims that it is low-fat or fat-free means that it has lower calorie content than the regular versions.
- Use the fat-free or low-fat version of salad dressing, mayonnaise, soft or liquid margarine, and vegetable oil. You can also use the regular versions but limit your consumption to half the amount you usually take.
- Choose low-fat or fat-free condiments
- Gradually cut back on the portions of your every meal.

Make it a Habit to Exercise

You can begin with a simple exercise program at the start of the diet if you are intent on maximizing the benefits of the DASH eating plan. You can try brisk walking for 15 minutes in the morning and at night. You can gradually shift to the more challenging exercises as your body gets used to the process.

Generally, doing a moderate-intensity exercise for 30 minutes each day is already beneficial to your health. If you have normal blood pressure but are not physically active, you'll have an increased risk of having high blood pressure when you get older or when you develop diabetes or when you become overweight.

If you are under medication for blood pressure, you can boost the effects of the medicines by doing moderate physical activity for 30 minutes each day. For people with moderately elevated blood pressure, you can do brisk walking for 30 minutes several times a week.

The DASH Eating Plan

This chart is essential in helping you follow this program. This is based on 1600 calories or 6500 kJ per day. You can add more or decrease the number of servings depending on how you normally eat. It is best to consult a dietitian about the number of servings most suitable for your age and health.

1. Fruits - sources of fiber, magnesium, and potassium. You can have them 4 times a day. One serving is equal to half a cup of frozen, canned or fresh fruit, 1/4 cup dried fruit, 1/2 cup fruit juice or 1 piece of fruit (medium-sized)

Samples of foods to eat:

- Frozen, dried or canned fruit and fruit juice
- Tangerine, strawberries, peach, raisin, orange, prune, pineapple, pear, apple, melon, mango, grape, date, banana, apricot

2. Vegetables - sources of fiber, magnesium, and potassium. You can have them 3 to 4 times a day. One serving is equal to half a cup of vegetable juice, half a cup of cooked vegetable or a cup of raw, leafy vegetable, such as spinach.

Samples of foods to eat:

- Unsalted or low sodium vegetable juice
- Turnip, tomato, squash, spinach, potato, pea, onion, leeks, kale, cucumber, celery, carrot, broccoli, beets, beans, artichoke

3. Grains and grain products - sources of fiber. You can have them 6 times a day. One serving is equal to half a cup of bulgur or couscous,

cereal, pasta, or rice, 1 ounce of dry cereal, 1/2 pita, bun, or bagel, or a slice of bread

Samples of foods to eat:

- Bulgur or couscous, whole wheat pasta, brown rice
- Whole grain cold or hot cereal
- Whole grain products - bread, bagel, pita, English muffin

4. Fats and oils - sources of healthy fats. You can have them twice a day. One serving is equal to 1 tablespoon of low-fat mayonnaise, 1 tablespoon margarine or 1 tablespoon vegetable oil

Samples of foods to eat:

- Low-fat mayonnaise
- Non-hydrogenated margarine
- Oils with high amounts of unsaturated fat - safflower, corn oil, canola, olive oil

5. Nuts, seeds, and legumes - sources of fiber, protein, potassium, and magnesium. You can have them thrice a week. One serving is equal to 2 tablespoons of peanut butter, half a cup of cooked legumes, 2 tablespoons of seeds or 1/3 cup of nuts

Samples of foods to eat:

- Lentils, chickpeas, kidney beans

- Unsalted sunflower seeds
- Unsalted peanut butter, hazelnuts, peanuts, walnuts, almonds

6. Fish, poultry, and meat - sources of magnesium and protein. You can have them twice a day. One serving is equal to 3 ounces of cooked fish, poultry or meat

Samples of foods to eat:

- Skinless chicken
- Boiled, roasted or broiled fish, poultry or meat
- Lean meat with the visible fat removed

7. Low-fat or non-fat milk products - sources of protein and calcium. You can have them 2 to 3 times a day. One serving is equal to 1 1/2 ounces of cheese, 1 cup yogurt or 1 cup milk.

Samples of foods to eat:

- Partly skimmed hard or light cheese
- Low-fat or non-fat yogurt
- One percent or skim milk

8. Sweets. You can have them 5 times or less each week. One serving is equal to a cup of lemonade, 5 jelly beans or 1 tablespoon of jelly jam or sugar

Samples of foods to eat:

- Low-fat sweets
- Sugar, sorbet, hard candy, fruit-flavored gelatin, jam, jelly, maple syrup

Sample of a DASH Eating Plan for One Week

The menus are based on the 2000 daily calorie intake. You can increase or decrease the serving size depending on your calorie requirement. The menus are also based on 2300 mg of daily sodium intake but there are certain ingredients with recommendations on how you can lower the sodium level to 1500 mg.

Day 1

Total number of calories per day - 2027 (2078 with substitutions)

Sodium level per day - 2035 mg (1560 mg with substitutions)

Breakfast

- 1 cup low-fat milk
- 1 medium banana
- 1 tablespoon peanut butter
- 1 mini whole wheat bagel

- 1/2 cup instant oatmeal (or 1/2 cup of regular oatmeal mixed with a teaspoon of cinnamon

Lunch

- 1 cup apple juice
- 1 cup cantaloupe chunks

Chicken breast sandwich with the following ingredients:

- 1 tablespoon low-fat mayonnaise
- 2 tomato slices
- 1 large leaf romaine lettuce
- 1 slice or 3/4 ounce natural reduced-fat cheddar cheese (or 1 slice or 3/4 ounce of natural low sodium Swiss cheese)
- 2 slices whole wheat bread
- 3 ounces skinless chicken breast

Dinner

- 1/2 cup canned pears with juice
- 1/2 cup cooked corn

Spinach salad with the following ingredients:

- 1 tablespoon vinaigrette salad dressing*
- 1/4 cup sliced fresh mushrooms
- 1/4 cup freshly grated carrots
- 1 cup spinach leaves

- 1 cup spaghetti
- 3 tablespoons Parmesan cheese
- 3/4 cup vegetarian spaghetti sauce* (substitute tomato paste in the recipe with low-sodium tomato paste)

Snacks

- 1 cup fat-free fruit yogurt (with no sugar added)
- 1/4 cup dried apricots
- 1/3 cup unsalted almonds

*Recipes:

Vinaigrette Salad Dressing

Serves: 4

Calories per serving: 33

Sodium per serving: 1 mg

Ingredients:

- 1/4 teaspoon black pepper
- 1 tablespoon virgin olive oil
- 1/4 teaspoon honey
- 1 tablespoon red wine vinegar
- 1/2 cup water
- 1 garlic bulb (separated and peeled)

Directions:

1. Put the garlic cloves in a pan over medium-high flame and add half a cup of water or just enough to cover all the pieces. Bring to a boil. Turn heat to low and simmer for 15 minutes or until tender.

2. Discard excess liquid, if needed, until the pan has about 2 tablespoons of liquid. Turn heat to high. Continue cooking for 3 minutes. Remove from the stove.

3. Sift the garlic and liquid to a bowl. Mash the garlic as you do this step.

4. Add vinegar to the bowl and whisk until combined. Add seasoning and oil and mix well.

Vegetarian Spaghetti Sauce

Serves: 6

Calories per serving: 105

Sodium per serving: 479 mg (253 mg after substitution)

Ingredients:

- 1 cup water
- 2 medium chopped tomatoes
- 1 6-ounce can tomato paste (substitute with low-sodium tomato paste)

- 1 8-ounce can tomato sauce
- 1 tablespoon dried basil
- 1 tablespoon dried oregano
- 1 1/4 cups sliced zucchini
- 3 garlic cloves (chopped)
- 2 onions (chopped)
- 2 tablespoons olive oil

Directions:

1. Heat oil in a pan over medium flame. Add garlic, onions, and zucchini. Cook for 5 minutes.

2. Stir in the rest of the ingredients. Cover the pan and simmer for 45 minutes.

3. Serve while warm with spaghetti.

Day 2

Total number of calories per day - 2101 (1507 with substitutions)

Sodium level per day - 2101 mg (1507 mg with substitutions)

Breakfast

- 1 cup orange juice
- 1 teaspoon soft tub margarine (or 1 teaspoon unsalted soft tub margarine)

- 1 slice whole wheat bread
- 1 cup low-fat milk
- 1 medium banana
- 3/4 cup bran flakes cereal (or 3/4 cup shredded wheat cereal)

Lunch

- 1/2 cup fruit cocktail with juice
- 1 tablespoon Dijon mustard (or 1 tablespoon regular mustard)
- 2 slices whole wheat bread
- 3/4 cup chicken salad* (do not use salt in the recipe)

Salad with the following ingredients:

- 1 teaspoon low-calorie Italian dressing
- 1 tablespoon sunflower seeds
- 1/2 cup tomato wedges
- 1/2 cup fresh cucumber slices

Dinner

- 1 cup low-fat milk
- 1 apple (small)
- 1 teaspoon soft tub margarine (or 1 teaspoon unsalted soft tub margarine)
- 1 small whole wheat roll
- 1 cup green beans (cooked in 1/2 teaspoon canola oil)

- 2 tablespoons fat-free beef gravy
- 3 ounces eye of the round beef

1 small baked potato with the following added ingredients:

- 1 tablespoon chopped scallions
- 1 tablespoon grated reduced-fat natural cheddar cheese (or 1 tablespoon low sodium, reduced-fat natural cheddar cheese)
- 1 tablespoon fat-free sour cream

Snacks

- 1 cup fat-free fruit yogurt (with no sugar added)
- 1/4 cup raisins
- 1/3 cup unsalted almonds

*Recipe:

Chicken Salad

Serves: 5

Calories per serving: 176

Sodium per serving: 179 mg (120 mg after omitting salt)

Ingredients:

- 3 tablespoons low-fat mayonnaise
- 1/8 teaspoon salt (or omit)
- 1/2 teaspoon onion powder
- 1 tablespoon lemon juice
- 1/4 cup chopped celery
- 3 1/4 cups skinless chicken breasts

Directions:

1. Put meat on a baking dish. Bake until cooked. Thinly slice and place in the fridge.

2. Put the chilled chicken in a bowl. Add the remaining ingredients and toss until combined.

Day 3

Total number of calories per day - 2124 (2045 with substitutions)

Sodium level per day - 2312 mg (1436 mg with substitutions)

Breakfast

- 1/2 cup grape juice
- 1 medium peach
- 1 cup fat-free fruit yogurt (with no sugar added)
- 1 teaspoon soft tub margarine (or 1 teaspoon unsalted soft tub margarine)

- 1 slice whole wheat bread

Lunch

- 1 cup carrot sticks

Ham and cheese sandwich with the following ingredients:

- 1 tablespoon low-fat mayonnaise
- 2 tomato slices
- 1 large leaf romaine lettuce
- 2 slices whole wheat bread
- 1 slice (3/4 ounce) reduced -fat natural cheddar cheese (or 1 slice (3/4 ounce) low sodium, reduced-fat natural cheddar cheese
- 2 ounces low sodium low-fat ham (or 2 ounces roast beef tenderloin)

Dinner

- 1 cup low-fat milk
- 1 cup cantaloupe chunks
- 1 cup green peas cooked in 1 teaspoon canola oil
- Chicken and Spanish Rice* (use low-sodium tomato sauce in the recipe)

Snacks

- 1 cup low-fat milk

- 1/4 cup apricots
- 1 cup apple juice
- 1/3 cup unsalted almonds

***Recipe:**

Chicken and Spanish Rice

Serves: 5

Calories per serving: 428

Sodium per serving: 341 mg (215 mg after substitution)

Ingredients:

- 3 1/2 cups skinless, boneless chicken breasts (cooked and diced)
- 5 cups cooked brown rice
- 1 1/4 teaspoons minced garlic
- 1/2 teaspoon back pepper
- 1 teaspoon chopped parsley
- 1 8-ounce can tomato sauce (substitute with 1 4-ounce can regular tomato sauce and 1 4-ounce can low-sodium tomato sauce)
- 2 teaspoons vegetable oil
- 3/4 cup green peppers
- 1 cup chopped onions

Directions:

1. Heat oil in a pan over medium flame. Add green peppers and onions and cook for 5 minutes.

2. Stir in the spices and tomato sauce. Cook for a couple of minutes. Add meat and rice and continue cooking until heated through.

Day 4

Total number of calories per day - 1997 (1995 with substitutions)

Sodium level per day - 2114 mg (1447 mg with substitutions)

Breakfast

- 1 cup orange juice
- 1 teaspoon soft tub margarine (or 1 teaspoon unsalted soft tub margarine)
- 1 slice whole wheat bread
- 1 cup low-fat milk
- 1 medium banana
- 3/4 cup bran flakes cereal (or 2 cups puffed wheat cereal)

Lunch

- 1 medium orange

- 1 cup New Potato Salad*

Beef barbecue sandwich with the following ingredients:

- 2 tomato slices
- 1 large leaf romaine lettuce
- 1 hamburger bun
- 2 slices (1 1/2 ounces) reduced-fat, natural cheddar cheese (or 1 1/2 low sodium, reduced-fat natural cheddar cheese)
- 1 tablespoon barbecue sauce
- 2 ounces eye of round beef

Dinner

- 1 small cornbread muffin cooked with 1 teaspoon soft tub margarine (or 1 teaspoon unsalted soft tub margarine)
- 1 cup spinach cooked with 1 tablespoon slivered almonds and 1 teaspoon canola oil
- 1/2 cup brown rice
- 3 ounces cod with 1 teaspoon lemon juice

Snacks

- 2 large graham crackers with 1 tablespoon peanut butter

- 1 tablespoon unsalted sunflower seeds
- 1 cup fat-free fruit yogurt (with no sugar added)

***Recipe:**

New Potato Salad

Serves: 5

Calories per serving: 196

Sodium per serving: 17 mg

Ingredients:

- 1 teaspoon dried dill weed
- 1/4 teaspoon black pepper
- 1/4 cup chopped green onions
- 2 tablespoons olive oil
- 16 small new potatoes

Directions:

1. Rinse the potatoes until thoroughly clean. Put in a pot and add enough water to cover them. Boil until tender. This will take about 20 minutes.

2. Drain water and leave potatoes for 20 minutes or until cool.

3. Cut each potato into 4 and place in a bowl. Add spices, onions, and olive oil. Toss until combined.

4. Place salad in the fridge and serve cold.

Day 5

Total number of calories per day - 1993 (1988 with substitutions)

Sodium level per day - 2069 mg (1421 mg with substitutions)

Breakfast

- 1 cup fat-free fruit yogurt (with no sugar added)
- 1 cup low-fat milk
- 1 medium banana
- 1 cup whole grain oat rings (or 1 cup regular oatmeal)

Lunch

- 1 cup low-fat milk
- 1 medium apple

Tuna salad sandwich with the following ingredients:

- 2 slices whole wheat bread
- 2 tomato slices
- 1 large leaf romaine lettuce
- 1 tablespoon low-fat mayonnaise
- 1/2 cup tuna (drained and rinsed)

Dinner

- 1 cup grape juice
- 1 teaspoon soft tub margarine (or 1 teaspoon unsalted soft tub margarine)
- 1 small whole wheat roll
- 1/6 of the Zucchini Lasagna recipe (follow substitutions)

Salad with the following ingredients:

- 1 tablespoon sunflower seeds
- 1 tablespoon reduced calorie vinaigrette dressing (or 1 tablespoon low-sodium vinaigrette dressing)
- 2 tablespoons seasoned croutons
- 1 cup tomato wedges
- 1 cup fresh spinach leaves

Snacks

- 6 whole wheat crackers
- 1/4 cup dry apricots
- 1/3 cup unsalted almonds

*Recipe:

Zucchini Lasagna

Serves: 6

Calories per serving: 200

Sodium per serving: 368 mg (165 mg after substitution)

Ingredients:

- 1/8 teaspoon black pepper
- 1 garlic clove
- 1/4 cup chopped onion
- 2 teaspoons dried oregano
- 2 teaspoons dried basil
- 2 1/2 cups low-sodium tomato sauce
- 1 1/2 cups sliced raw zucchini
- 1/4 cup grated Parmesan cheese
- 1 1/2 cups fat-free cottage cheese (substitute with low sodium, fat-free cottage cheese)
- 3/4 cup grated part-skim mozzarella cheese
- 1/2 pound cooked lasagna noodles

Directions:

1. Put a tablespoon of Parmesan cheese and 1/8 cup mozzarella cheese in a bowl. Mix until combined. Set aside.

2. Put the cottage cheese in another bowl. Add the remaining Parmesan and mozzarella cheese. Mix until combined and set aside.

3. Put the tomato sauce in a bowl and add the rest of the ingredients. Mix well.

4. Lightly spray a baking dish with vegetable oil. place a thin layer on the bottom and spread all over. Arrange 1/3 of the cooked noodles on top, followed by the cottage cheese mixture and a layer of zucchini. Spread a thin layer of the sauce topped with the noodles and the reserved cheese mixture.

5. Cover the dish with a foil. Bake in a preheated oven at 350 degrees F for 40 minutes.

6. Allow to cool before slicing into 6.

Day 6

Total number of calories per day - 1976 (2100 with substitutions)

Sodium level per day - 2373 mg (1519 mg with substitutions)

Breakfast

- 1 cup orange juice
- 1 tablespoon peanut butter (or 1 tablespoon unsalted peanut butter)
- 1 medium raisin bagel
- 1 cup low-fat milk
- 1 medium banana
- 1 cup whole grain oat rings cereal (or 1 cup frosted shredded wheat)

Lunch

Cucumber salad with the following ingredients:

- 1 tablespoon unsalted almonds
- 1/2 cup canned pineapple
- 1/2 cup low-fat cottage cheese
- 1 tablespoon vinaigrette dressing (or 2 tablespoons fat-free yogurt dressing*)
- 1/2 cup tomato wedges
- 1 cup fresh cucumber slices

Tuna salad plate with the following ingredients:

- 1 slice whole wheat bread
- 1 large leaf romaine lettuce
- 1/2 cup Tuna Salad*

Dinner

- 1 medium peach
- 1 small whole wheat roll

- 1 cup collard greens cooked with 1 teaspoon canola oil
- 3 ounces Turkey Meatloaf* (follow substitutions in the recipe)

1 small baked potato with the following:

- 1 chopped scallion stalk
- 1 tablespoon grated reduced-fat natural cheddar cheese (or 1 tablespoon low sodium, reduced-fat natural cheddar cheese)
- 1 tablespoon fat-free sour cream

Snacks

- 2 tablespoons unsalted sunflower seeds
- 1 cup fat-free fruit yogurt (with no sugar added)

*Recipes:

Yogurt Salad Dressing

Serves: 5

Calories per serving: 39

Sodium per serving: 66 mg

Ingredients:

- 2 tablespoons lemon juice
- 2 tablespoons dried dill
- 2 tablespoons dried chives
- 1/4 cup low-fat mayonnaise
- 8 ounces fat-free plain yogurt

Directions:

1. Put all ingredients in a bowl. Mix well. Refrigerate until ready to serve.

Tuna Salad

Serves: 5

Calories per serving: 138

Sodium per serving: 171 mg

Ingredients:

- 6 1/2 tablespoons low-fat mayonnaise
- 1/3 cup chopped green onions
- 1/2 cup chopped raw celery
- 2 6-ounce cans tuna (packed in water)

Directions:

1. Drain and rinse tuna. Place in a bowl and use a fork to break it apart. Add mayonnaise, onion, and celery. Mix until combined.

Turkey Meatloaf

Serves: 5

Calories per serving: 191

Sodium per serving: 205 mg (74 mg after substitution)

Ingredients:

- 1/4 cup ketchup (use low-sodium ketchup)
- 1 tablespoon dehydrated onion flakes
- 1 large egg
- 1/2 cup dry regular oats
- 1 pound lean ground turkey

Directions:

1. Put all ingredients in a bowl. Mix until combined. Transfer to a loaf pan.

2. Bake in a preheated oven at 350 degrees F for 25 minutes.

3. Leave until slightly cool before slicing into 5.

Day 7

Total number of calories per day - 1939 (1935 with substitutions)

Sodium level per day - 1671 mg (1472 mg with substitutions)

Breakfast

- 1 cup low-fat milk
- 1 cup orange juice
- 1/2 cup fat-free fruit yogurt (with no sugar added)
- 1 medium banana
- 1 low-fat granola bar

Lunch

- 1 medium orange
- 1 cup steamed broccoli
- Turkey breast sandwich with the following ingredients:
- 1 tablespoon Dijon mustard (or 1 tablespoon regular mustard)
- 2 teaspoons low-fat mayonnaise
- 2 tomato slices
- 1 large leaf romaine lettuce
- 2 slices whole wheat bread
- 3 ounces turkey breast

Dinner

- 1 small cookie
- 1 teaspoon soft tub margarine
- 1 small whole wheat roll

- 1 cup cooked carrots
- 1 cup Scallion Rice*
- 3 ounces Spicy Baked Fish*

Sautéed spinach with the following ingredients:

- 1 tablespoon unsalted slivered almonds
- 2 teaspoons canola oil
- 1/2 cup spinach

Snacks

- 1/4 cup dried apricots
- 1 cup low-fat milk
- 2 tablespoons unsalted peanuts

*Recipes:

Scallion Rice

Serves: 5

Calories per serving: 200

Sodium per serving: 18 mg

Ingredients:

- 1/4 cup chopped scallions or green onions
- 1 1/2 teaspoons low-sodium bouillon granules
- 4 1/4 cups cooked brown rice

Directions:

1. Cook rice according to package directions.

2. Put the cooked rice in a bowl. Add the bouillon granules and scallions. Mix until combined.

Spicy Baked Fish

Serves: 4

Calories per serving: 192

Sodium per serving: 50 mg

Ingredients:

- 1 teaspoon salt-free spicy seasoning
- 1 tablespoon olive oil
- 1 pound fish fillet (salmon)

Directions:

1. Rinse fish. Place in paper towels to remove excess moist. Transfer to a baking dish. Rub with oil and seasoning.

2. Bake in a preheated oven at 350 degrees F for 15 minutes. Divide into 4 and serve along with rice.

Chapter 2 – Appetizer Recipes

Corn Relish with Black Bean

Serves: 8

Calories per serving: 112

Sodium per serving: 93 mg

Ingredients:

- 1 lemon (juiced)
- 2 teaspoon sugar
- 1 red bell pepper (seeded and diced)
- 1/2 cup fresh parsley (chopped)
- 1/2 cup red onion (diced)
- 2 garlic cloves (chopped)
- 3 cups diced tomatoes
- 1 cup frozen corn kernels (thawed)
- 1 15.5-ounce can black beans (rinsed and drained)

Directions:

1. Put all ingredients in a bowl. Toss until combined. Cover the bowl and keep in the fridge for at least half an hour before serving.

Tomato Crostini

Serves: 4

Calories per serving: 107

Sodium per serving: 176 mg

Ingredients:

- 1/4 pound crusty Italian peasant bread (sliced into 4)
- Freshly ground pepper
- 1 garlic clove (minced)
- 2 teaspoons olive oil
- 1/4 cup fresh basil (minced)
- 4 plum tomatoes (chopped)

Directions:

1. Put basil, tomatoes, pepper, and garlic in a bowl. Toss until combined. Cover the bowl and leave at room temperature for 30 minutes.

2. Toast the bread slices. Top with the tomato mixture and serve at once.

Healthy Greens and Artichoke Dip

Serves: 8

Calories per serving: 78

Sodium per serving: 130 mg

Ingredients:

- 1/2 cup sour cream (low-fat)
- 2 tablespoons Parmesan cheese (grated)
- 1 cup unsalted white beans (prepared)
- 1 tablespoon freshly minced parsley (or 1 teaspoon dried parsley)
- 1 teaspoon freshly minced thyme (or 1/3 teaspoon dried thyme)
- 1 teaspoon ground black pepper
- 2 garlic cloves (minced)
- 4 cups raw spinach (chopped)
- 1 15.5-ounce can artichoke hearts in water (drained)

Directions:

1. Put all the ingredients in a bowl. Mix until combined. Transfer to a baking dish. Bake in a preheated oven at 350 degrees F for half an hour.

2. Serve while warm.

Tortilla Crisps with Fruity Salsa

Serves: 8

Calories per serving: 105

Sodium per serving: 181 mg

Ingredients:

For the salsa:

- 2 tablespoons orange juice
- 1 tablespoon honey (or agave nectar)
- 2 tablespoons sugar-free jam (any flavor of your choice)
- 3 cups diced fresh fruits of choice

For the tortilla:

- 1/2 tablespoon cinnamon
- 1 tablespoon sugar
- Cooking spray
- 8 whole wheat fat-free tortillas (sliced into 8 wedges)

Directions:

1. Combine sugar and cinnamon in a bowl.

2. Arrange tortilla wedges in 2 baking sheets. Lightly spray with the cooking spray. Sprinkle with the cinnamon and sugar mixture. Bake in a preheated oven at 350 degrees F for 12 minutes. Leave to cool.

3. Put orange juice, honey, and jam in a bowl. Mix well. Add the diced fruits. Gently toss to coat. Cover the bowl and keep in the fridge for 3 hours.

4. Top chips with salsa before serving.

Chicken Polenta

Serves: 8 (2 wedges per serving)

Calories per serving: 157

Sodium per serving: 160 mg

Ingredients:

For the topping:

- 2 tablespoons minced flat-leaf parsley
- 2 tablespoons grated Parmesan cheese
- 1/4 cup dry-packed sun-dried tomatoes (rehydrate by soaking in water, drain, and chop)
- 1/4 cup pitted Kalamata olives (chopped)
- 1/2 yellow onion (minced)
- 1/2 tablespoon extra-virgin olive oil

For the polenta:

- 3 egg whites
- 1/4 teaspoon freshly ground black pepper
- 1 teaspoon dry mustard
- 1 tablespoon chopped thyme (you can use basil or oregano)
- 3 garlic cloves (chopped)
- 1/2 tablespoon extra-virgin olive oil

- 1 cup chicken or vegetable stock (or broth)
- 2 cups plain soy milk
- 1 3/4 cups chickpea flour

Directions:

1. Prepare the batter. Put mustard, thyme, garlic, pepper, olive oil, stock, soy milk, and flour in a food processor. Process until combined and smooth. Transfer to a bowl and refrigerate for an hour.

2. Beat the egg whites using an electric mixer until stiff peaks form. Gradually fold the egg whites in the cooled batter. Transfer to a lightly greased baking pan. Bake in a preheated oven at 425 degrees F for 15 minutes. Leave to cool.

3. Prepare the topping. Heat oil in a pan over medium-high flame. Add onion and cook for 6 minutes or until golden brown. Stir in tomatoes and olives. Cook for a minute. Remove from the stove.

4. Put the cooked onion mixture on the baked polenta and spread evenly. Top with cheese. Broil for a minute or until lightly browned. Place on a wire rack. Add parsley on top and leave for 10 minutes to cool.

5. Slice and serve.

Tasty Grilled Mushrooms

Serves: 4

Calories per serving: 65

Sodium per serving: 15 mg

Ingredients:

- 1 tablespoon fresh basil (chopped)
- 2 tablespoons fresh ginger (peeled and chopped)
- 1/2 cup pineapple juice
- 1/4 cup balsamic vinegar
- 4 large portobello mushrooms (remove the stems)

Directions:

1. Put ginger, pineapple juice, and vinegar in a bowl. Whisk until combined.

2. Use a damp cloth to clean the mushrooms. Arrange them in a glass dish with the stemless part facing up. Drizzle marinade on top and cover the dish. Keep in the fridge for 30 minutes, flip the mushrooms and put back in the fridge for 30 more minutes.

3. Put the marinated mushrooms on a lightly greased grill. Cook each side for 5 minutes. Turn them often during cooking while basting with the marinade to keep them moist.

4. Transfer cooked mushrooms to a platter, top with basil and serve at once.

Potato Skins Bites

Serves: 2

Calories per serving: 50

Sodium per serving: 12 mg

Ingredients:

- 1/8 teaspoon freshly ground black pepper
- 1 tablespoon fresh rosemary (minced)
- Butter-flavored cooking spray
- 2 medium russet potatoes

Directions:

1. Rinse potatoes until clean. Pierce each piece using a fork. Bake in a preheated oven at 375 degrees F for an hour or until the skins are crisp.

2. Carefully transfer potatoes to a cutting board. Divide each piece into 2. Scoop the pulp out while leaving about 1/8 inch of the flesh. Save pulp for another recipe.

3. Lightly grease the inner part of the potato skin with the cooking spray. Season with

pepper and rosemary. Bake for 10 minutes and serve while hot.

Artichoke with Spinach Dip

Serves: 8

Calories per serving: 123

Sodium per serving: 114 mg

Ingredients:

- 1/2 cup sour cream (reduced-fat)
- 2 tablespoons grated Parmesan cheese
- 1 cup white beans (cooked)
- 1 tablespoon freshly minced parsley
- 2 garlic cloves (minced)
- 1 teaspoon dried thyme (minced)
- 4 cups spinach (chopped)
- 1 tablespoon black pepper
- 2 cups artichoke hearts

Directions:

1. Put the beans in a food processor and process until pureed. Transfer to a bowl. Add the rest of the ingredients. Mix until combined.

2. Transfer the mixture to a baking dish. Bake in a preheated oven at 350 degrees for 30 minutes.

3. You can serve this dip along with crackers, whole grain bread or slices of vegetables.

Mushrooms Filled with Basil Pesto

Serves: 20

Calories per serving: 59

Sodium per serving: 80 mg

Ingredients:

- 20 crimini mushrooms (rinsed and stems removed)

For the filling:

- 1/2 teaspoon kosher salt
- 2 teaspoons lemon juice
- 1 tablespoon fresh garlic
- 2 tablespoons pumpkin seeds
- 1/4 cup Parmesan cheese
- 2 cups fresh basil leaves

For the topping:

- 3 tablespoons fresh parsley (chopped)
- 1/4 cup melted butter

- 1 1/2 cups panko breadcrumbs

Directions:

1. Arrange mushrooms caps faced upside-down on a baking sheet.

2. Prepare the topping. In a bowl, put parsley, butter, and breadcrumbs. Mix well.

3. Prepare the filling. Put lemon juice, garlic, salt, oil, pumpkin seeds, cheese, and basil in a food processor. Process until combined.

4. Scoop filling in each mushroom cap and add a teaspoon of the topping. Gently pat the topping down using the back of a spoon. Bake in a preheated oven at 350 degrees F for 15 minutes.

Dried Chickpea Hummus

Serves: 6

Calories per serving: 116

Sodium per serving: 210 mg

Ingredients:

- 1 teaspoon ground cumin
- 3 tablespoons fresh cilantro (chopped)
- 2 tablespoons sherry vinegar

- 3/4 cup, plus 2 tablespoons spring onion (sliced)
- 1 tablespoon olive oil
- 1/2 teaspoon salt
- 1 bay leaf
- 2 garlic cloves
- 3 cups water
- 2/3 cup dried chickpeas

Directions:

1. Rinse chickpeas and soak in water overnight. Drain the following day.

2. Put chickpeas in a pan over high flame. Add water, 1/4 teaspoon of salt, bay leaf, and garlic cloves. Bring to a boil. Partially cover the pan and turn heat to low. Simmer for an hour or until the beans are tender.

3. Discard bay leaf. Reserve the garlic and half of the cooking liquid. Drain the rest of the liquid.

4. Put vinegar, 1/4 teaspoon of salt, cumin, cilantro, 3/4 cup spring onion, olive oil, cooked garlic, and chickpeas in a food processor. Process until pureed. Add a tablespoon of the cooking liquid at a time until the consistency is similar to a thick spread.

5. Transfer mixture to a bowl and top with the remaining onions. Serve at once.

Fruity Kebabs

Serves: 2 (2 kebabs per serving)

Calories per serving: 190

Sodium per serving: 53 mg

Ingredients:

- 4 red grapes
- 1/2 banana (chunked)
- 1 kiwi (peeled and cut into 4)
- 4 strawberries
- 4 pineapple chunks
- 1 teaspoon lime zest
- 6 ounces low-fat lemon yogurt (sugar-free)

Directions:

1. Prepare the dip. Put lime zest, lime juice, and yogurt in a small bowl. Whisk until combined. Cover the bowl and keep in the fridge until ready to use.

2. Prepare 4 wooden skewers. Thread a piece of each fruit variety in a skewer.

3. Serve kebabs along with the prepared dip.

Shrimp with Chipotle

Serves: 4

Calories per serving: 109

Sodium per serving: 139 mg

Ingredients:

- 1/2 teaspoon fresh oregano (chopped)
- 1/2 teaspoon chipotle chili powder
- 1/2 teaspoon minced garlic
- 1/2 teaspoon extra-virgin olive oil
- 1 1/2 teaspoons water
- 2 tablespoons tomato paste
- 1 pound shrimp (peeled and deveined)

Directions:

1. Put shrimp in a bowl of cold water. Drain and transfer to paper towels to dry.

2. Prepare the marinade. Put oil, water, tomato paste, oregano, chili powder, and garlic in a small bowl. Whisk until combined. Spread all over the shrimp. Cover and keep in the fridge for at least an hour.

3. Thread shrimp on skewers or put them in a grill basket. Put on a lightly greased grill and cook each side for 4 minutes or until done.

4. Serve while warm.

Spicy Avocado Dip

Serves: 4

Calories per serving: 85

Sodium per serving: 57 mg

Ingredients:

- 1/2 cup mashed ripe avocado
- 1/8 teaspoon hot sauce
- 2 teaspoons onion (chopped)
- 1/2 cup sour cream (fat-free)

Directions:

1. Put all ingredients in a bowl and mix until combined.

2. You can serve this as dipping for sliced veggies or baked tortilla chips.

Breaded Shrimp

Serves: 6 (2 pieces per serving)

Calories per serving: 75

Sodium per serving: 396 mg

Ingredients:

- 12 large shrimp (peeled and deveined)
- 1/2 cup coconut milk
- 1/2 teaspoon kosher salt
- 1/4 cup panko breadcrumbs
- 1/4 cup sweetened coconut

Directions:

1. Put coconut milk in a small bowl.

2. Put breadcrumbs, coconut, and salt in a food processor. Process until combined. Transfer to a bowl.

3. Dip shrimp in coconut milk before coating with the panko mixture. Arrange the coated pieces on a lightly greased baking sheet.

4. Bake in a preheated oven at 375 degrees F for 15 minutes.

Wrapped Brie and Cranberry

Serves: 12

Calories per serving: 116

Sodium per serving: 133 mg

Ingredients:

- 1 egg white
- 2 tablespoons water

- 6 ounces Brie cheese (cubed)
- 1 sheet puff pastry dough (cut into 12 squares)
- 1 cinnamon stick
- 2 tablespoons sugar
- 1/2 medium orange (cut into 4)
- 1/2 cup cranberries (fresh or frozen)

Directions:

1. Heat a bit of oil in a pan over medium-high flame. Turn heat to low before putting orange, cranberries, cinnamon stick, and sugar. Cook for 10 minutes while constantly stirring. Turn off the heat. Discard the orange quarters and cinnamon stick. Leave to cool.

2. Place the pastry dough on a flat surface. Put a teaspoon of the cranberry mixture and one cube of cheese in each square.

3. Mix water and egg whites in a small bowl. Dab a bit of the mixture on the sides of the inner part of the pastry dough using a brush. Fold the dough to envelop the filling. Brush the surface of the pastry with the egg mixture.

4. Arrange pastry squares on a baking dish. Bake in a preheated oven at 425 degrees F for 12 minutes.

Baba Ghanoush

Serves: 4

Calories per serving: 233

Sodium per serving: 150 mg

Ingredients:

- 2 rounds of whole wheat pita
- Black pepper to taste
- 1 tablespoon olive oil
- 1 tablespoon fresh basil (chopped)
- 1 lemon (juiced)
- 1 red bell pepper (cut in half and seeded)
- 2 eggplants (cut lengthwise and peeled)
- 1 garlic bulb (cut the top off)

Directions:

1. Heat on side of a greased grill. Wrap garlic bulb in foil and place on the cooler side of the grill. Cook for 30 minutes.

2. Put bell pepper and eggplant slices on the hot part of the grill. Cook each side for 3 minutes.

3. Get roasted cloves from the garlic bulb and put in a food processor. Add pepper, olive oil, basil, lemon juice, and grilled bell pepper and eggplant. Process until smooth. Transfer to a bowl.

4. Grill bread for a couple of seconds or until warm. Serve along with the dip.

Chapter 3 – Breakfast Recipes

Healthy Oatmeal

Serves: 1

Calories per serving: 345

Sodium per serving: 53 mg

Ingredients:

- 2 tablespoons toasted walnuts (chopped)
- 1/2 cup fresh fruits of choice
- 1 tablespoon honey
- 3 tablespoons plain yogurt (reduced-fat)
- 3 tablespoons fat-free milk
- 1/3 cup old-fashioned oats

Directions:

1. Put oats in a mason jar. Add honey, yogurt, and milk. Mix until combined. Put nuts and fruits on top. Cover the jar and leave in the fridge overnight.

You can tweak the recipe by using other ingredients to give your oatmeal different flavors. Here are some of the flavors you can try to include:

- Banana bread oats – Use maple syrup instead of honey. Add half a teaspoon of cinnamon and half of a mashed banana. Mix well and place toasted pecans on top.
- Choco-cherry oats – Use a tablespoon of cocoa powder and mix with cherry-flavored yogurt. Add frozen pitted of fresh cherries on top.
- Pina colada oats – Mash half of a banana and mix it with the oat mixture along with a tablespoon of shredded coconut and 2 tablespoons of crushed pineapple.

Note:

You can prepare this recipe several days in advance. If you want to omit dairy, replace yogurt or milk with half a cup of coconut milk or soy milk.

Power Sweet Potato Breakfast

Serves: 4

Calories per serving: 321

Sodium per serving: 36 mg

Ingredients:

- 1/4 cup unsweetened coconut flakes (toasted)
- 2 tablespoons maple syrup
- 1 medium apple (chopped)
- 1/2 cup coconut Greek yogurt (fat-free)
- 4 medium sweet potatoes

Directions:

1. Arrange potatoes on a baking sheet lined with tin foil. Bake in a preheated oven at 400 degrees F for 45 minutes to 1 hour.

2. Cut the top of each potato with an X mark. Use a fork to fluff the top.

3. Place the rest of the ingredients on top of each baked potato.

Note:

You can tweak the toppings depending on your preference. If you don't have an oven and you want to cook the potatoes in a microwave, scrub the skin first before piercing each piece using a form. Put the potatoes on a heatproof plate before cooking in the microwave, uncovered, for 6 minutes. Flip them and cook for 6 more minutes. Add a couple of minutes cooking time if needed or until the veggies are tender.

Fruity Granola

Serves: 4

Calories per serving: 340

Sodium per serving: 88 mg

Ingredients:

- 2 tablespoons honey
- 2 tablespoons sunflower kernels
- 2 tablespoons sliced almonds (toasted)
- 1/2 cup granola (without raisins)
- 1 cup fresh raspberries
- 2 small peaches (sliced)
- 2 cups fat-free vanilla Greek yogurt
- 4 small bananas (peeled and halved lengthwise)

Directions:

1. Toast the almonds. Spread them in a pan and bake for 5 minutes at 350 degrees F. Flip the nuts and continue baking for 5 more minutes or until lightly browned.

2. Prepare 4 shallow dishes and put the same amount of bananas in each. Put the rest of the ingredients on top.

Quinoa with Peppers

Serves: 4

Calories per serving: 261

Sodium per serving: 760 mg

Ingredients:

- 1/8 teaspoon salt
- 1/4 teaspoon pepper
- 1/4 teaspoon garam masala
- 1 garlic clove (minced)
- 3/4 cup chopped sweet onion
- 1 medium green pepper (chopped)
- 1 medium sweet red pepper (chopped)
- 1 pound Italian turkey sausage links (casings removed)
- 3/4 cup quinoa (rinsed)
- 1 1/2 cups vegetable stock

Directions:

1. Put the stock in a saucepan over medium-high flame. Bring to a boil before adding quinoa. Turn the heat to low and cover the pan. Simmer for 15 minutes or until the liquid is fully absorbed. Turn off the flame.

2. Heat a skillet over medium-high flame. Add the onion and sausage. Crumble meat as you cook for 10 minutes. Stir in the seasonings and

garlic. Cook for a minute and add the cooked quinoa.

Note:

You can cook quinoa in advance. Let it cool and put in an airtight container. Store in the freezer. Partially thaw overnight before preparing. Place in a heat-proof container, cover, and reheat in the microwave on a high while occasionally stirring.

Bow Ties and Beans

Serves: 4

Calories per serving: 348

Sodium per serving: 394 mg

Ingredients:

- 1/2 cup crumbled feta cheese
- 3/4 teaspoon freshly ground pepper
- 1 2-ounce can sliced ripe olives (drained)
- 1 15-ounce can cannellini beans (rinsed and drained)
- 2 large tomatoes (chopped)
- 2 garlic cloves (minced)
- 1 medium zucchini (sliced)
- 1 tablespoon olive oil

- 2 1/2 cups uncooked whole wheat bow tie pasta

Directions:

1. Check package about how to cook your pasta. Reserve half a cup of cooking water and drain the rest.

2. Put oil in a pan over medium-high flame. Once heated, add zucchini to the pan and cook for 4 minutes or until crisp. Stir in garlic and cook for 30 seconds. Add pepper, olives, beans, and tomatoes. Turn the heat to low and simmer for 5 minutes while occasionally stirring.

3. Add pasta and enough of the reserved water to get it moist. Add cheese and gently mix until combined.

Minty Chickpea Tabbouleh

Serves: 4

Calories per serving: 380

Sodium per serving: 450 mg

Ingredients:

- 1/4 teaspoon pepper
- 1/2 teaspoon salt
- 2 tablespoons lemon juice

- 2 tablespoons julienned soft sun-dried tomatoes
- 1/4 cup olive oil
- 1/4 cup minced fresh mint
- 1/2 cup minced fresh parsley
- 1 15-ounce can chickpeas or garbanzo beans (rinsed and drained)
- 1 cup fresh or frozen peas (thawed)
- 2 cups water
- 1 cup bulgur

Directions:

1. Put water and bulgur in a pan over medium-high flame and bring to a boil. Turn heat to low, cover the pan and simmer for 10 minutes. Add peas, stir and cover the pan. Turn the heat to low and simmer for 5 minutes or until the peas and bulgur are cooked.

2. Put the cooked dish in a bowl and add the rest of the ingredients.

3. You can serve it warm or keep in the fridge and eat it cold.

Chickpea and Sweet Potato Pitas

Serves: 6

Calories per serving (2 pita halves with filling): 462

Sodium per serving: 662 mg

Ingredients:

- 1/4 cup fresh cilantro (minced)
- 12 whole wheat pita pocket halves (warmed)
- 2 cups arugula or baby spinach
- 1 teaspoon ground cumin
- 1 tablespoon lemon juice
- 1 cup plain Greek yogurt
- 2 garlic cloves (minced)
- 1/2 teaspoon salt (divided)
- 2 teaspoons garam masala
- 3 tablespoons canola oil (divided)
- 1 medium red onion (chopped)
- 2 15-ounce cans chickpeas or garbanzo beans (rinsed and drained)
- 2 medium sweet potatoes (peeled and cubed)

Directions:

1. Put the potatoes in a heatproof container. Microwave for 5 minutes on high.

2. Add onion, chickpeas, 1/4 teaspoon of salt, garam masala, and 2 tablespoons of oil to the potatoes. Toss until combined. Transfer to a baking pan and spread all over.

3. Roast in a preheated oven at 400 degrees F for 15 minutes. Leave to cool.

4. Put the rest of the oil and garlic in a heatproof bowl. Microwave on high for a minute or until the garlic is lightly browned. Add the rest of the salt, cumin, lemon juice, and yogurt. Mix well.

5. Put arugula in a bowl. Add the potato mixture and mix well. Scoop mixture into pitas and drizzle with sauce. Sprinkle with cilantro on top.

Potato and Bean Rice Bowls

Serves: 4

Calories per serving: 435

Sodium per serving: 405 mg

Ingredients:

- 2 tablespoons sweet chili sauce
- 1 15-ounce can black beans (rinsed and drained)

- 4 cups chopped fresh kale (discard tough stems)
- 1 medium red onion (finely chopped)
- 1 large sweet potato (peeled and diced)
- 3 tablespoons olive oil (divided)
- 1 1/2 cups water
- 1/4 teaspoon garlic salt
- 3/4 cup uncooked long-grain rice
- Additional sweet chili sauce (optional)
- Lime wedges (optional)

Directions:

1. Put water, garlic salt, and rice in a pan over medium-high flame. Bring to a boil. Cover the pan and turn the heat to low. Simmer for 20 minutes or until the rice is tender. Turn off the heat and leave for 5 minutes.

2. Put 2 tablespoons of oil in a pan over medium-high flame. Once the oil is heated, add the sweet potato and sauté for 8 minutes. Stir in the onion and cook for 6 minutes or until the potato is tender. Add kale and continue cooking for 5 minutes. Add beans and stir for a couple of minutes.

3. Transfer the cooked rice to a bowl. Add the rest of the oil and gradually add 2 tablespoons of chili sauce. Mix well. Gently stir in the potato mixture.

4. Serve while warm. Add lime wedges and more chili sauce, if desired.

Nutty Chai Granola

Serves: 8 cups

Calories per serving (1/2 cup): 272

Sodium per serving: 130 mg

Ingredients:

- 1/4 teaspoon ground cardamom
- 3/4 teaspoon ground nutmeg
- 3/4 teaspoon ground cinnamon
- 3/4 teaspoon salt
- 2 teaspoons vanilla extract
- 1/3 cup sugar
- 1/4 cup olive oil
- 1/2 cup honey
- 1 cup sweetened shredded coconut
- 2 cups almonds (coarsely chopped)
- 3 cups quick-cooking oats
- 1/4 cup boiling water
- 2 chai tea bags

Directions:

1. Put boiling water in a cup and steep tea bags for 5 minutes.

2. Put coconut, almonds, and oats in a bowl. Mix until combined.

3. Discard the tea bags and add the rest of the ingredients to the tea. Pour over the oat mixture. Mix well. Transfer to a lightly oiled baking pan. Bake in a preheated oven at 250 degrees F for an hour and 15 minutes or until golden brown while stirring every 20 minutes.

4. Leave to cool. Put in an airtight container and leave in the fridge until ready to serve.

Banana Pancakes

Serves: 8

Calories per serving (2 pancakes): 186

Sodium per serving: 392 mg

Ingredients:

- 1/2 teaspoon vanilla extract
- 1 tablespoon maple syrup
- 1 tablespoon olive oil
- 2/3 cup mashed ripe banana
- Additional syrup and banana slices (optional)
- 2 cups fat-free milk
- 2 large eggs
- 1/2 teaspoon salt

- 1 teaspoon ground cinnamon
- 4 teaspoons baking powder
- 1 cup all-purpose flour
- 1 cup whole wheat flour

Directions:

1. In a bowl, put salt, ground cinnamon, baking powder, and all-purpose flour. Whisk until combined.

2. In another bowl, put vanilla, a tablespoon of syrup, oil, mashed banana, milk, and eggs. Mix well. Gradually add to the flour mixture while whisking.

3. Preheat a lightly greased pan over medium flame. Cook 1/4 cup of the batter for every pancake. Cook until both sides are browned. Cook the rest of the batter.

4. You can serve the pancakes with additional syrup and sliced bananas on top.

Note:

You can cook the pancakes in advance or store leftovers. First, make sure they are cooled. Put the pieces in between sheets of waxed paper before putting inside a Ziploc bag. Freeze until ready to use.

To reheat, put the frozen pancakes on a baking sheet. Cover with foil and heat in the oven for 15 minutes at 375 degrees F. You can also heat

2 pancakes at a time in the microwave. Put them in a heatproof plate and microwave for 60 seconds on high.

Peach and Berry Pancake

Serves: 4

Calories per serving: 199

Sodium per serving: 149 mg

Ingredients:

- 1/4 cup vanilla yogurt
- 1/2 cup all-purpose flour
- 1/8 teaspoon salt
- 1/2 cup fat-free milk
- 3 large eggs (lightly beaten)
- 1 tablespoon butter
- 1/2 cup fresh raspberries
- 1/2 teaspoon sugar
- 2 medium peaches (peeled and sliced)

Directions:

1. Put the raspberries, peaches, and sugar in a bowl. Gently toss to coat.

2. Put milk, eggs, and salt in a bowl. Whisk until combined. Gradually add flour as you whisk.

3. Place butter in a pie plate and melt in a preheated oven at 400 degrees F for 3 minutes. Remove from the oven and spread melted butter all over. Add the batter and bake for 22 minutes or until browned and puffed.

4. Top with yogurt and mixed fruits.

Cheese and Black Bean Frittata

Serves: 6

Calories per serving: 183

Sodium per serving: 378 mg

Ingredients:

- 1 cup canned black beans (rinsed and drained)
- 2 garlic cloves (minced)
- 3 green onions (finely chopped)
- 1/3 cup sweet red pepper (finely chopped)
- 1/3 cup green pepper (finely chopped)
- 1/2 cup white cheddar cheese (shredded)
- 1 tablespoon olive oil
- 1/4 teaspoon pepper
- 1/4 teaspoon salt
- 1 tablespoon fresh parsley (minced)

- 1/4 cup salsa
- 3 large egg whites
- 6 large eggs
- Optional toppings: additional salsa, sliced ripe olives, and minced fresh cilantro

Directions:

1. Put the eggs, egg whites, pepper, salt, parsley, and salsa in a bowl. Whisk until combined.

2. Heat oil in a skillet over medium-high flame. Stir in green onions and peppers. Cook until tender or about 4 minutes. Add garlic and continue cooking for a minute. Add beans and mix well. Turn heat to medium before adding the egg mixture. Give it a quick stir and cook until slightly set. Add cheese on top.

3. Put skillet about 4 inches from heat in a preheated broiler. Broil for 4 minutes or until browned.

4. Leave for 5 minutes before slicing into wedges.

5. Top with any topping of choice before serving.

Cabbage Roll Skillet

Serves: 6

Calories per serving: 332

Sodium per serving: 439 mg

Ingredients:

- 4 cups cooked brown rice
- 1 medium green pepper (cut into thin strips)
- 1 small head cabbage (thinly sliced)
- 1/2 teaspoon pepper
- 1 teaspoon dried thyme
- 1 teaspoon dried oregano
- 1 tablespoon brown sugar
- 2 tablespoons cider vinegar
- 1 8-ounce can tomato sauce
- 1 large onion (chopped)
- 1 pound extra-lean ground beef (95 percent lean)
- 1 28-ounce can whole plum tomatoes (chop the tomatoes and reserve the liquid)

Directions:

1. Preheat a skillet over medium-high flame. Put beef and onion and cook for 8 minutes whole breaking meat into crumbles. Add the

reserved liquid, tomatoes, seasonings, brown sugar, vinegar, and tomato sauce. Mix well.

2. Add pepper and cabbage. Cover the skillet and cook for 6 minutes while occasionally stirring. Remove the cover and continue cooking for 8 minutes.

3. Serve dish with rice.

Cheesy Tortilla Wrap

Serves: 1

Calories per serving: 319

Sodium per serving: 444 mg

Ingredients:

- 1 whole wheat tortilla, warmed
- 1 green onion (chopped)
- 1 teaspoon butter
- 4 fresh asparagus spears (trimmed and sliced)
- 1/8 teaspoon pepper
- 2 teaspoons grated Parmesan cheese
- 1 tablespoon fat-free milk
- 2 large egg whites
- 1 large egg

Directions:

1. Put egg, egg whites, pepper, cheese, and milk in a bowl. Whisk until combined.

2. Lightly grease a skillet over medium flame. Put the asparagus and cook until crisp or about 4 minutes. Transfer to a plate.

3. Add butter to the same skillet and turn heat to medium-high. Once butter is melted, add the egg mixture. Push the sides of the egg in the middle part as it starts to cook. Once thickened, add asparagus and green onion on either side of the egg and fold it in half.

4. Serve omelet with warm tortilla.

Portobello Mushrooms Florentine

Serves: 2

Calories per serving: 126

Sodium per serving: 472 mg

Ingredients:

- 1/4 cup goat or feta cheese (crumbled)
- 1/8 teaspoon salt
- 2 large eggs
- 1 cup fresh baby spinach
- 1 small onion (chopped)

- 1/2 teaspoon olive oil
- 1/8 teaspoon pepper
- Minced fresh basil (optional)
- 1/8 teaspoon garlic salt
- Cooking spray
- 2 large Portobello mushrooms (stems removed)

Directions:

1. Arrange mushrooms in a lightly greased baking pan with the stem side facing up. Spritz with a bit of cooking spray and sprinkle with pepper and garlic salt. Bake in a preheated oven at 425 degrees F for 10 minutes or until tender.

2. Heat oil in a skillet over medium-high flame. Put onion and cook for 3 minutes. Add spinach and stir until wilted.

3. Put eggs and salt in a bowl and whisk until combined. Add to the skillet and cook until eggs are done. Turn off the heat.

4. Scoop the cooked egg mixture to the mushrooms. Add cheese and basil on top.

Note:

You can tweak the recipe by trying other fillings, such as goat cheese with garbanzos and quinoa; tomatoes, basil and feta; or sauce, cooked sausage, and mozzarella.

Chapter 4 – Main Course Recipes

Herbed Pork Roast

Serves: 8

Calories per serving: 289

Sodium per serving: 326 mg

Ingredients:

- 1/2 teaspoon salt
- 3 tablespoons cornstarch
- 1 teaspoon grated orange zest
- 1 tablespoon soy sauce (reduced-sodium)
- 1 tablespoon steak sauce
- 1 tablespoon white grapefruit juice
- 1 tablespoon sugar
- Minced fresh oregano (optional)
- Egg noodles (cooked)
- 1 cup, plus 3 tablespoons orange juice
- 2 medium onions, sliced into thin wedges
- 1/2 teaspoon pepper
- 1/2 teaspoon ground ginger
- 1 teaspoon dried oregano

- 1 boneless pork sirloin roast (cut in half)

Directions:

1. In a bowl, put pepper, ginger, and oregano. Mix well. Rub mixture all over the meat.

2. Heat a greased skillet over medium-high flame. Put roast and cook until all sides are browned. Transfer to a slow cooker. Stir in onions.

3. Put soy sauce, steak sauce, grapefruit juice, sugar, and a cup of orange juice in a bowl. Mix well. Pour over the meat. Cover slow cooker and cook for 5 hours on low setting.

4. Scoop out onions and meat and place on a plate. Discard fat from the cooking liquid. Transfer to a pan over medium-high flame. Add salt and orange zest.

5. In a small bowl, mix the rest of the orange juice and cornstarch until combined. Gradually add to the pan as you stir. Cook for a couple of minutes or until thick. Remove from heat.

6. Serve noodles and pork along with the sauce. Top with fresh oregano.

Garlic Chicken with White Wine

Serves: 4

Calories per serving: 243

Sodium per serving: 381 mg

Ingredients:

- 1/2 cup reduced-sodium chicken broth or dry white wine
- 2 garlic cloves (minced)
- 1 medium onion (chopped)
- 2 cups sliced baby Portobello mushrooms
- 1 tablespoon olive oil
- 1/4 teaspoon pepper
- 1/2 teaspoon salt
- 4 chicken breast halves (boneless and skinless)

Directions:

1. Pound with mallet until the thickness is about 1/2 inches. Season with pepper and salt.

2. Heat oil in a pan over medium flame. Add meat and cook each side for 6 minutes. Transfer to a plate and loosely cover with foil.

3. Put onion and mushrooms to the pan and turn heat to medium-high. Cook until tender. Stir in garlic and cook for a minute. Add wine.

Stir the sides and bottom of the pan and bring to a boil. Cook for a couple of minutes or until the liquid is reduced.

4. Pour sauce over chicken and serve.

Sautéed Kale with Creamy Lentils

Serves: 4

Calories per serving: 321

Sodium per serving: 661 mg

Ingredients:

- 2 cups brown or basmati rice (cooked)
- 2 tablespoons grated Romano cheese
- 1/2 teaspoon Italian seasoning
- 3 garlic cloves (minced)
- 1 14-ounce can water-packed artichoke hearts (drained and chopped)
- 16 cups fresh kale (chopped)
- 1 tablespoon grapeseed oil or olive oil
- 1/4 teaspoon sea salt (divided)
- 1 1/4 cups vegetable broth
- 1/8 teaspoon pepper
- 1/4 teaspoon dried oregano
- 1/2 cup dried red lentils (rinsed and sorted)

Directions:

1. Put vegetable broth in a saucepan over medium-high flame. Add lentils, oregano, and pepper. Bring to a boil. Cover the pan and simmer for 15 minutes. Turn off the heat.

2. Heat oil in a stockpot over medium heat. Stir in kale and the rest of the salt. Cover the pot and cook for 5 minutes while stirring every now and then. Add the Italian seasoning and artichoke hearts. Cook for 3 minutes. Turn off the heat, add cheese and stir until combined. Serve over rice.

Spiced Sole Fillets

Serves: 4

Calories per serving: 174

Sodium per serving: 166 mg

Ingredients:

- 2 green onions (thinly sliced)
- 1 medium tomato (chopped)
- 1/8 teaspoon cayenne pepper
- 1/4 teaspoon lemon-pepper seasoning
- 1/4 teaspoon paprika
- 4 sole fillets
- 2 garlic cloves (minced)

- 2 cups fresh mushrooms (sliced)
- 2 tablespoons butter

Directions:

1. Melt butter in a pan over medium-high flame. Stir in mushrooms and garlic. Cook until tender. Add the fillets and season with cayenne, lemon pepper, and paprika. Cover the pan and cook for 10 minutes. Add green onions and tomato.

Tasty Salmon

Serves: 8

Calories per serving: 403

Sodium per serving: 153 mg

Ingredients:

- 1 salmon fillet
- 1/4 teaspoon dill weed
- 1/2 teaspoon pepper
- 1/2 teaspoon paprika
- 1/2 teaspoon ground mustard
- 1/2 teaspoon garlic powder
- 1 tablespoon olive oil
- 1 tablespoon butter (melted)
- 1 tablespoon soy sauce

- 2 tablespoons packed brown sugar
- A dash of cayenne pepper
- A dash of dried tarragon
- A dash of salt

Directions:

1. Put all ingredients, except salmon, together in a bowl. Mix well. Rub mixture all over salmon. Transfer to a greased grill rack, cover and cook for 15 minutes of medium heat.

Salmon Fillets with Nutty Crust

Serves: 6

Calories per serving: 376

Sodium per serving: 219 mg

Ingredients:

- 1 garlic clove (minced)
- 1/4 teaspoon red pepper flakes (crushed)
- 1/2 teaspoon grated orange or lemon zest
- 1 tablespoon snipped fresh dill
- 2 tablespoons prepared horseradish
- 2 tablespoons olive oil
- 1/2 cup minced shallots

- 2/3 cup chopped pistachios
- 2/3 cup dry bread crumbs
- 1/3 cup sour cream
- 6 salmon fillets

Directions:

1. Put fish in a baking pan with the skin side facing down. Brush each fillet with sour cream.

2. In a bowl, put the rest of the ingredients and mix until combined. Put on top of the fillets. Press using your hands to make the coating stick to the fish. Bake in a preheated oven at 350 degrees F for 15 minutes.

Grilled Tilapia with Salsa

Serves: 8

Calories per serving: 131

Sodium per serving: 152 mg

Ingredients:

- 1/8 teaspoon pepper
- 8 tilapia fillets
- 1 tablespoon canola oil
- A dash cayenne pepper
- 1/8 teaspoon, plus 1/4 teaspoon salt

- 4 teaspoons, plus 2 tablespoons lime juice
- 1/4 cup fresh cilantro (minced)
- 1/4 cup green pepper (finely chopped)
- 2 green onions (chopped)
- 2 cups fresh pineapple (cubed)

Directions:

1. Prepare the salsa. In a bowl, put cayenne, 1/8 teaspoon salt, 4 teaspoons lime juice, cilantro, green pepper, green onions, and pineapple. Mix well. Refrigerate until ready to serve.

2. In a bowl, mix the rest of the lime juice and oil. Pour on top of the fillets. Add the rest of the salt and pepper.

3. Put the fish on a griller, cover and grill each side for 3 minutes over medium heat.

4. Serve fish along with the prepared salsa.

Chicken Pasta Skillet

Serves: 6

Calories per serving: 403

Sodium per serving: 432 mg

Ingredients:

- 1 cup Thai peanut sauce
- 2 cups shredded cooked chicken
- 2 cups julienned carrots
- Chopped fresh cilantro (optional)
- 1 medium cucumber (cut into 2 lengthwise and sliced diagonally)
- 1 10-ounce package fresh sugar snap peas (trimmed and cut into thin strips)
- 2 teaspoons canola oil
- 6 ounces uncooked whole wheat spaghetti

Directions:

1. Cook spaghetti according to what's indicated in the package directions. Drain liquid.

2. Heat oil in a pan over medium-high flame. Add carrots and snap peas and cook for 8 minutes. Add spaghetti, peanut sauce, and meat. Toss until combined.

3. Transfer cooked dish to a plate. Top with cilantro and cucumber.

Pork Chops Curry

Serves: 6

Calories per serving: 478

Sodium per serving: 475 mg

Ingredients:

- 4 cups brown rice (cooked)
- 2 tablespoons almonds (toasted and slivered)
- 1/2 teaspoon chili powder
- 1/2 teaspoon salt
- 2 teaspoons curry powder
- 4 teaspoons sugar
- 1 28-ounce can whole tomatoes (undrained)
- 3 medium apples (thinly sliced)
- 1 small onion (minced)
- 6 boneless pork loin chops
- 4 teaspoons butter (divided)

Directions:

1. Melt 2 teaspoons of butter in a stockpot over medium-high flame. Cook meat in batches until browned. Transfer to a plate.

2. Add the rest of the butter to the same stockpot. Set heat to medium. Cook onion for 3 minutes. Add chili powder, salt, curry powder, sugar, tomatoes, and apples. Stir and bring to a boil. Put the meat back to the pot. Turn heat to low and simmer for 5 minutes. Flip the meat and cook for 5 more minutes. Turn off the heat and leave for 5 minutes.

3. Serve along with rice and add chopped almonds on top.

Penne Pasta with Beef

Serves: 4

Calories per serving: 532

Sodium per serving: 434 mg

Ingredients:

- 1/4 cup crumbled Gorgonzola cheese
- 1/4 cup walnuts (chopped)
- 1/3 cup prepared pesto
- 2 cups grape tomatoes (halved)
- 6 cups fresh baby spinach (coarsely chopped)
- 1/4 teaspoon pepper
- 1/4 teaspoon salt
- 2 beef tenderloin steaks
- 2 cups whole wheat penne pasta (uncooked)

Directions:

1. Cook pasta according to the indicated directions in its package. Drain liquid and put pasta in a bowl. Add walnuts, pesto, tomatoes, and spinach. Toss until combined.

2. Season meat with salt and pepper. Put on a grill over medium heat and cover. Cook each side for 7 minutes. Thinly slice and add to the pasta. Top with cheese before serving.

Beans and Tomato Pasta

Serves: 8

Calories per serving: 275

Sodium per serving: 429 mg

Ingredients:

- 3 cups baby spinach or arugula
- 1/2 teaspoon pepper
- 1 teaspoon minced fresh rosemary
- 1 teaspoon salt
- 3 garlic cloves (minced)
- Chopped fresh parsley (optional)
- 1 tablespoon olive oil
- 2 tablespoons fresh basil (minced)
- 1/4 cup grated Parmesan cheese
- 1/2 cup part-skim ricotta cheese
- 1/2 cup red onion (finely chopped)
- 1 cup fresh or frozen corn (thawed)
- 2 cups cherry tomatoes (halved)
- 1 15-ounce can cannellini beans (rinsed and drained)

- 3 cups whole wheat elbow macaroni (uncooked)

Directions:

1. Cook pasta according to the indicated directions in the package. Drain liquid. Rinse with cold water and drain.

2. Put pepper, rosemary, salt, garlic, oil, basil, Parmesan cheese, ricotta cheese, onion, corn, tomatoes, and beans in a bowl. Mix well. Pour over the pasta along with arugula. Gently toss until coated.

3. Top with parsley before serving.

Orzo Pasta with Shrimp

Serves: 4

Calories per serving: 406

Sodium per serving: 307 mg

Ingredients:

- 1/2 cup crumbled feta cheese
- 1/4 teaspoon pepper
- 2 tablespoons minced fresh cilantro
- 1 1/4 pounds uncooked shrimp (peeled and deveined)
- 2 tablespoons lemon juice

- 2 medium tomatoes (chopped)
- 2 garlic cloves (minced)
- 2 tablespoons olive oil
- 1 1/4 cups whole wheat orzo pasta (uncooked)

Directions:

1. Cook orzo according to the directions indicated in its package. Drain liquid.

2. Heat oil in a pan over medium flame. Cook garlic for a minute. Add lemon juice and tomatoes. Bring to a boil. Stir in shrimp. Turn heat to low and simmer for 5 minutes. Add pepper, cilantro, and cooked orzo. Stir until heated through.

3. Transfer to a bowl and top with feta cheese.

Chapter 5 – Salad Recipes

Tomato Salad with Turkey

Serves: 6

Calories per serving: 351

Sodium per serving: 458 mg

Ingredients:

- 3 medium tomatoes (chopped)
- 1 tablespoon fresh basil (thinly sliced)
- 1/4 cup chopped red onion
- 1 celery rib (coarsely chopped)
- 1 medium green pepper (coarsely chopped)
- 1/4 teaspoon salt
- 1/4 teaspoon dried oregano
- 1/2 teaspoon sugar
- 1 tablespoon red wine vinegar
- 2 tablespoons olive oil

For the turkey:

- 3 tablespoons olive oil
- 1/4 teaspoon pepper
- 1/4 teaspoon salt
- 1 20-ounce package turkey breast tenderloins

- 1 teaspoon lemon-pepper seasoning
- 1/2 cup finely chopped walnuts
- 1/2 cup grated Parmesan cheese
- 1 cup panko bread crumbs
- 2 tablespoons lemon juice
- 1 large egg
- Fresh basil as toppings

Directions:

1. Prepare the salad. Put salt, dried oregano, sugar, red wine vinegar, and olive oil in a bowl. Whisk until combined. Add basil, onion, celery, tomatoes, and green pepper. Mix well.

2. Whisk egg and lemon juice in another bowl.

3. Put lemon pepper, walnuts, cheese, and bread crumbs in a shallow container. Mix well.

4. Cut tenderloins in slices with an inch thickness. Use a meat mallet to flatten the slices into half its original thickness. Season with salt and pepper.

5. Soak each slice of meat in the egg mixture before coating with the crumb mixture.

6. Heat a tablespoon of oil in a pan over medium-high flame. Put 1/3 of the coated turkey slices. Cook until both sides are browned. Continue the process until you're done with all the coated turkey slices.

7. Serve turkey along with tomato salad. Top with basil before serving.

Salad Greens with Shredded Pork

Serves: 12

Calories per serving: 233

Sodium per serving: 321 mg

Ingredients:

- 1 cup corn (fresh or frozen)
- 1 small red onion (chopped)
- 2 medium tomatoes (chopped)
- 1 15-ounce can black beans (rinsed and drained)
- 12 cups mixed salad greens (torn)
- 1/2 teaspoon dried oregano
- 1/2 teaspoon ground cumin
- 1 cup shredded part-skim mozzarella cheese
- 1 teaspoon pepper
- 1 teaspoon chili powder
- 1 1/2 teaspoons hot pepper sauce
- Salad dressing of your choice
- 1 1/2 teaspoons salt
- 3 garlic cloves (minced)

- 1 4-ounce can green chilies (drained and chopped)
- 1 1/2 cups apple cider or juice
- 1 boneless pork loin roast

Directions:

1. Mix oregano, cumin, pepper, chili powder, pepper sauce, salt, garlic, green chilies, and cider in a bowl.

2. Put pork in a slow cooker and pour the seasoning mixture on top. Cover the cooker and cook for up to 8 hours on low.

3. Transfer cooked pork to a platter and shred meat using 2 forks.

4. Place salad greens on a bowl. Add shredded meat, cheese, corn, onion, tomatoes, and black beans on top. Add salad dressing before serving.

Note:
You can cook shredded pork in advance. Place in a container and cover the pieces with cooking juices. Cover container and store in the freezer. When ready to use, place in the refrigerator overnight to partially thaw. Put in a saucepan and mix until heated through.

Grilled Steak Salad

Serves: 4

Calories per serving: 456

Sodium per serving: 378 mg

Ingredients:

- 2 large tomatoes (coarsely chopped)
- 2 cups uncooked multigrain bow tie pasta
- 1 tablespoon olive oil
- 1 large sweet onion (cut into 1/2-inch rings)
- 2 large ears sweet corn (husked and cut from cob)
- 3 poblano peppers (halved, seeded, and chopped)
- 1/4 teaspoon pepper
- 1/4 teaspoon ground cumin
- 1/4 teaspoon salt
- 1 beef top sirloin steak

For the dressing:

- 1/3 cup chopped fresh cilantro
- 1/4 teaspoon pepper
- 1/4 teaspoon ground cumin
- 1/4 teaspoon salt
- 1 tablespoon olive oil
- 1/4 cup lime juice

Directions:

1. Season steak with pepper, cumin, and salt. Brush onion, corn, and poblano peppers with oil.

2. Cover steak as you grill over medium flame up to 8 minutes or until you have achieved your preferred doneness. Cut into thin slices.

3. Cover veggies as you grill up to 10 minutes or until crisp but tender. Flip them every once in a while.

4. Prepare the dressing. Put pepper, cumin, cilantro, salt, oil, and lime juice in a bowl. Mix well.

5. Put the veggies in a bowl.

6. Cook pasta according to the directions indicated in its package. Transfer to the bowl with veggies. Add dressing and toss until coated. Add meat and serve at once.

Steak and Berry Salad

Serves: 4

Calories per serving: 289

Sodium per serving: 452 mg

Ingredients:

- 2 tablespoons lime juice
- 2 teaspoons olive oil
- 1/4 teaspoon pepper
- 1/2 teaspoon salt
- 1 beef top sirloin steak

For the salad:

- 1/4 cup chopped walnuts (toasted)
- 1/4 cup crumbled blue cheese
- 1/4 cup red onion (thinly sliced)
- Reduced-fat balsamic vinaigrette
- 2 cups fresh strawberries (halved)
- 1 bunch romaine, torn

Directions:

1. Rub meat with pepper and salt. Heat oil in a pan over medium flame. Cook each side of meat up to 7 minutes. Transfer to a plate and leave for 5 minutes. Cut into small strips and add lime juice.

2. Place onion, strawberries, and romaine on a platter. Add steak, walnuts, and cheese. Drizzle with vinaigrette before serving.

Thai Cobb Salad

Serves: 6

Calories per serving: 382

Sodium per serving: 472 mg

Ingredients:

- 2 tablespoons creamy peanut butter
- 3/4 cup Asian toasted sesame salad dressing
- 1/4 cup fresh cilantro leaves
- 1/2 cup unsalted peanuts
- 1 cup fresh snow peas (halved)
- 1 medium sweet red pepper (julienned)
- 1 medium carrot (shredded)
- 1 medium ripe avocado (peeled and thinly sliced)
- 3 hard-boiled large eggs (coarsely chopped)
- 2 cups rotisserie chicken (shredded)
- 1 bunch romaine (torn)

Directions:

1. Arrange romaine in a platter. Add cilantro, peanuts, veggies, avocado, eggs, and chicken.

2. Put peanut butter and salad dressing in a bowl. Whisk until combined. Serve salad along with the sauce.

Quinoa and Zucchini Salad

Serves: 4

Calories per serving: 310

Sodium per serving: 353 mg

Ingredients:

- 1/4 teaspoon pepper
- 2 tablespoons fresh basil (minced)
- 1/4 cup Greek olives (finely chopped)
- 1/2 cup crumbled feta cheese
- 1 medium tomato (finely chopped)
- 3/4 cup canned garbanzo beans or chickpeas (rinsed and drained)
- 2 cups water
- 1 medium zucchini (chopped)
- 2 garlic cloves (minced)
- 1 cup quinoa (rinsed and well drained)
- 1 tablespoon olive oil

Directions:

1. Heat oil in a pan over medium-high flame. Put garlic and quinoa and cook for 3 minutes while constantly stirring. Add water and zucchini. Bring to a boil. Turn heat to low and cover the pan. Cook until most liquid is gone or about 15 minutes. Add the rest of the ingredients and stir until heated through.

Pintos Salad with Warm Rice

Serves: 4

Calories per serving: 331

Sodium per serving: 465 mg

Ingredients:

- 1/4 cup cheddar cheese (finely shredded)
- 1 bunch romaine (quartered lengthwise through the core)
- 1/4 cup fresh cilantro (chopped)
- 1/2 cup salsa
- 1 4-ounce can green chilies (chopped)
- 1 8.8-ounce package ready-to-serve brown rice
- 1 15-ounce can pinto beans (rinsed and drained)
- 1 1/2 teaspoons ground cumin
- 1 1/2 teaspoons chili powder
- 2 garlic cloves (minced)
- 1 small onion (chopped)
- 1 cup frozen corn
- 1 tablespoon olive oil

Directions:

1. Heat oil in a pan over medium-high flame. Put onion and corn and cook for 5 minutes. Add cumin, chili powder, and garlic. Cook for a minute as you stir. Add cilantro, salsa, green

chilies, rice, and beans. Cook until heated through.

2. Arrange romaine wedges on a plate. Add the cooked rice and beans and sprinkle with cheese.

Shrimp and Corn Salad

Serves: 4

Calories per serving: 371

Sodium per serving: 450 mg

Ingredients:

- 1 pound uncooked shrimp (peeled and deveined)
- 1 medium ripe avocado (peeled and chopped)
- 1/8 teaspoon pepper
- 1 1/2 cups cherry tomatoes (halved)
- 1/2 teaspoon salt (divided)
- 1/4 cup olive oil
- 1/2 cup packed fresh basil leaves
- 4 medium ears sweet corn (husked)

Directions:

1. Cook corn in a pot of boiling water until tender. Drain water and leave to cool. Cut from cob and put in a bowl.

2. Put 1/4 teaspoon of salt, oil, and basil in a food processor. Process until blended.

3. Add the rest of the salt, pepper, 2 tablespoons of basil mixture, avocado, and tomatoes to the corn. Toss until combined.

4. Put shrimp in skewers. Baste with the rest of the basil mixture. Grill each side for 4 minutes over medium heat. Remove from the skewers and add to the salad.

Lentil Salad

Serves: 8

Calories per serving: 225

Sodium per serving: 404 mg

Ingredients:

- 1 cup crumbled feta cheese
- 4 cups fresh baby spinach (chopped)
- 1 teaspoon dried oregano
- 1 teaspoon dried basil
- 2 teaspoons honey
- 3 tablespoons olive oil

- 4 cooked and crumbled bacon strips (optional)
- 1/4 cup fresh mint (minced)
- 1/2 cup rice vinegar
- 1/2 cup chopped soft sun-dried tomato halves
- 1 small red onion (chopped)
- 1 medium zucchini (cubed)
- 1 medium cucumber (cubed)
- 2 cups sliced fresh mushrooms
- 2 cups water
- 1 cup dried lentils (rinsed)

Directions:

1. Put water and lentils in a pan over medium-high flame. Bring to a boil. Turn heat to low, cover the pan and simmer for 25 minutes. Drain liquid and immediately soak in cold water to rinse. Drain all moisture before transferring to a bowl.

2. Add tomatoes, onion, zucchini, cucumber, and mushrooms to the salad.

3. Put oregano, basil, honey, oil, mint, and vinegar in a small bowl and whisk. Pour over the salad and toss until coated. Add bacon, cheese, and spinach. Gently toss before serving.

Edamame Salad

Serves: 6

Calories per serving: 317

Sodium per serving: 355 mg

Ingredients:

- 1/2 cup sesame ginger salad dressing
- 2 green onions (diagonally sliced)
- 1/2 cup salted peanuts
- 1 cup fresh bean sprouts
- 3 clementine (peeled and segmented)
- 2 cups frozen shelled edamame (thawed)
- 1 15-ounce can garbanzo beans or chickpeas (rinsed and drained)
- 6 cups baby kale salad blend

Directions:

1. Put all salad ingredients together. Drizzle with sauce and toss until combined.

Shrimp and Greens Salad

Serves: 4

Calories per serving: 252

Sodium per serving: 448 mg

Ingredients:

- 1 tablespoon minced fresh tarragon
- 1 1/2 teaspoons honey
- 1 1/2 teaspoons Dijon mustard
- 3 tablespoons cider vinegar
- 1/3 cup orange juice

For the salad:

- 1/2 cup red onion (finely chopped)
- 1 cup grape tomatoes (halved)
- 2 medium nectarines (cut into smaller pieces)
- 8 cups mixed salad greens (torn)
- 1/4 teaspoon salt
- 1/2 teaspoon lemon-pepper seasoning
- 1 pound uncooked shrimp (peeled and deveined)
- 1 cup fresh or frozen corn
- 4 teaspoons canola oil (divided)

Directions:

1. In a bowl, put honey, mustard, vinegar, and orange juice. Mix well. Add tarragon and mix until combined.

2. Heat a teaspoon of oil in a pan over medium-high flame. Put corn and cook for a couple of minutes or until tender. Transfer to a bowl.

3. Put remaining oil in the pan where you cooked the corn. Set heat to medium-high. Add

shrimp. Season with salt and lemon pepper. Cook for 4 minutes. Turn off the heat, add corn and stir. Transfer to a bowl.

4. Put the rest of the ingredients in another bowl, add 1/3 cup of the dressing and gently toss until combined. Add the cooked shrimp and corn. Serve with the rest of the dressing.

Chapter 6 – Dessert and Beverage Recipes

Rice Pudding with Mango

Serves: 4

Calories per serving: 275

Sodium per serving: 176 mg

Ingredients:

- 1 teaspoon vanilla extract
- 1/2 teaspoon ground cinnamon
- 2 tablespoons sugar
- 1 cup vanilla soy milk
- Peeled and chopped mango (optional)
- 1 medium ripe mango (peeled, sliced, and mashed)
- 1 cup long-grain brown rice (uncooked)
- 1/4 teaspoon salt
- 2 cups water

Directions:

1. Put water and salt in a pan over medium-high flame. Bring to a boil. Add rice. Turn heat to low and cover the pan. Simmer for 40 minutes. Add mashed mango, cinnamon,

sugar, and milk. Continue cooking for 15 minutes while occasionally stirring.

2. Turn off the heat and add vanilla.

3. You can have this hot or cold. Top with chopped mango, if preferred, before serving.

Light Choco Pudding

Serves: 4

Calories per serving: 127

Sodium per serving: 112 mg

Ingredients:

- 1 teaspoon vanilla extract
- 2 cups chocolate soy milk
- 1/8 teaspoon salt
- 2 tablespoons baking cocoa
- 2 tablespoons sugar
- 3 tablespoons cornstarch

Directions:

1. Put milk in a pan over medium flame. Add salt, cocoa, sugar, and cornstarch. Mix until thick and bubbly. Turn heat to low and continue cooking for 2 minutes.

2. Turn off the heat, add vanilla and allow to cool while stirring every now and then. Transfer to a bowl, cover and refrigerate for 30 minutes before serving.

Peach Tart

Serves: 8

Calories per serving: 222

Sodium per serving: 46 mg

Ingredients:

- 1 cup all-purpose flour
- 1/4 teaspoon ground nutmeg
- 3 tablespoons sugar
- 1/4 cup butter (softened)

For the filling:

- 1/4 cup sliced almonds
- 1/8 teaspoon almond extract
- 1/4 teaspoon ground cinnamon
- Whipped cream (optional)
- 2 tablespoons all-purpose flour
- 1/3 cup sugar
- 2 pounds peaches (peeled and sliced)

Directions:

1. Put butter, sugar, and butter in a bowl. Mix until fluffy. Add flour and beat until combined. Transfer to a tart pan and firmly spread and press to the bottom. Put on a baking sheet in the oven's middle rack. Bake in a preheated oven at 375 degrees F for 12 minutes. Leave to cool.

2. Put peaches in a bowl. Add almond extract, cinnamon, flour, and sugar. Toss to coat. Scoop on top of the crust. Add chopped almonds on top. Put on the lower rack of the oven and bake for 40 minutes. Allow to cool.

3. Serve as is or you cal also opt to top it with whipped cream.

Yogurt Parfait with Lime and Grapefruit

Serves: 6

Calories per serving: 207

Sodium per serving: 115 mg

Ingredients:

- 3 tablespoons honey
- 2 tablespoons lime juice
- 2 teaspoons grated lime zest
- Fresh mint leaves (torn)

- 4 cups plain yogurt (reduced-fat)
- 4 large red grapefruit

Directions:

1. Cut a small part of each grapefruit's top and bottom. Make them stand on a cutting board. Cut off peel and gently slice through the membrane of the fruit's segment to get the fruit.

2. Put juice, lime zest, and yogurt in a bowl. Arrange half of the grapefruit in 6 parfait glasses. Top each glass with half of the yogurt mixture. Repeat until you have no more fruit and yogurt mixture left. Top each glass with honey and mint.

Fruit and Nut Bites

Serves: 4 dozen

Calories per serving (1 piece): 86

Sodium per serving: 15 mg

Ingredients:

- 1 cup pistachios (toasted and finely chopped)
- 1 cup dried cherries (finely chopped)
- 2 cups dried apricots (finely chopped)
- 1/4 cup honey

- 1/4 teaspoon almond extract
- 3 3/4 cups sliced almonds (divided)

Directions:

1. Put 1 1/4 cups of almonds in a food processor. Pulse until chopped. Transfer to a bowl and set aside.

2. Process 2 1/2 cups almonds in a food processor until chopped. Gradually add extract and honey as you process. Transfer to a bowl. Add cherries and apricots. Divide into 6 and shape them into thick rolls. Wrap in plastic and leave in the fridge for an hour.

3. Remove plastic and cut each roll to 1 1/2 inch piece. Roll half of them in pistachios. Roll the other half in almonds. Wrap each piece in waxed paper and store in an airtight container.

Grilled Pineapple

Serves: 6

Calories per serving: 97

Sodium per serving: 35 mg

Ingredients:

- 1 1/2 teaspoons chili powder
- 1 tablespoon honey
- 1 tablespoon olive oil

- A dash salt
- 1 tablespoon lime juice
- 3 tablespoons brown sugar
- 1 fresh pineapple (peeled, cored and cut into 6 wedges)

Directions:

1. Prepare the glaze. Put all ingredients, except the pineapple, in a bowl. Mix until combined. Brush fruit with half of the mixture and reserve the rest.

2. Put the coated pineapple in a griller over medium heat. Cover and grill each side for 4 minutes. Baste every now then with the remaining glaze.

Pumpkin Cake with Hazelnut

Serves: 8

Calories per serving: 166

Sodium per serving: 73 mg

Ingredients:

- 2 eggs (lightly beaten)
- 3 tablespoons firmly packed brown sugar
- 1/2 cup honey

- 3/4 cup canned pumpkin puree (homemade or unsweetened)
- 3 tablespoons canola oil
- 1/2 teaspoon ground nutmeg
- 1/2 teaspoon ground cinnamon
- 1/2 teaspoon ground allspice
- 1/2 teaspoon baking powder
- 2 tablespoons flaxseed
- 1/2 cup all-purpose flour
- 1 cup whole-wheat flour
- 2 tablespoons chopped hazelnuts
- 1/4 teaspoon salt
- 1/4 teaspoon ground cloves

Directions:

1. Put eggs, brown sugar, canola oil, honey, and pumpkin puree in a bowl. Whisk using an electric mixer on low speed.

2. Put all flour, salt, cloves, nutmeg, cinnamon, allspice, baking powder, and flaxseed in another bowl. Whisk until combined. Add to the pumpkin mixture. Beat until blended.

3. Transfer batter to a lightly greased loaf pan. Sprinkle hazelnuts on top. Gently press to slightly dip the nuts in the batter. Bake in a preheated oven at 350 degrees F for 55 minutes. Leave on a wire rack to cool. Unmold and allow to cool completely.

4. Slice and serve.

Grapes with Sour Cream Sauce

Serves: 6

Calories per serving: 106

Sodium per serving: 32 mg

Ingredients:

- 3 tablespoons chopped walnuts
- 1 1/2 cups green seedless grapes
- 1 1/2 cups red seedless grapes
- 1/8 teaspoon vanilla extract
- 1/2 teaspoon lemon juice
- 1/2 teaspoon lemon zest
- 2 tablespoons powdered sugar
- 1/2 cup fat-free sour cream

Directions:

1. Put powdered sugar, sour cream, vanilla, lemon juice, and lemon zest in a bowl. Whisk until combined. Cover the bowl and chill for at least 4 hours.

2. Put grapes in 6 dessert bowls or glasses. Scoop sauce on top and add half a tablespoon of chopped walnuts in each cup.

3. Serve at once.

Angel Food Cake

Serves: 6

Calories per serving: 180

Sodium per serving: 214 mg

Ingredients:

- 6 tablespoons water
- 1/2 cup sugar
- 3/4 cup chopped rhubarb
- 1 1/2 cup strawberries (chopped)
- 3/4 cup reduced-fat whipped topping
- 1 pre-made angel food cake (sliced into 6 pieces)
- 1/8 teaspoon cinnamon
- 1 3/4 teaspoons vanilla

Directions:

1. Prepare the sauce. Put water, cinnamon, vanilla, sugar, rhubarb, and strawberries in a pan over medium flame. Stir for 5 minutes or before it boils. Turn off the heat and set aside.

2. Broil or grill angel food cake until all sides are browned. This will take about 3 minutes. Divide into serving plates. Put 2 tablespoons of the whipped topping and 1/4 cup of the strawberry sauce in each serving.

Grilled Fruit with Syrup

Serves: 4

Calories per serving: 208

Sodium per serving: 9 mg

Ingredients:

- 1/2 cup balsamic vinegar
- 2 tablespoons brown sugar
- Butter-flavored cooking spray
- Mint or basil leaves for garnish
- 2 large peaches (cored and cut in half)
- 2 large mangoes (cored and cut in half)
- 1 small pineapple (peeled, cored and sliced into 4 wedges)

Directions:

1. Put peaches, mangoes, and pineapple in a bowl. Coat with cooking spray as you toss the fruit pieces. Add brown sugar and toss until combined.

2. Put vinegar in a pan over low flame. Simmer as you stir until the liquid is reduced in half. Turn off the heat.

3. Broil or grill coated fruits for 5 minutes over medium heat. Transfer to serving plates. Scoop

vinegar on top and add basil or mint as garnishing.

Fruits with Cream Cheese

Serves: 4

Calories per serving: 201

Sodium per serving: 241 mg

Ingredients:

- 4 tablespoons shredded coconut (toasted)
- 1 8-ounce can water-packed pineapple chunks (drained)
- 1 14.5-ounce can water-packed sliced peaches (drained)
- 1 15-ounce can mandarin oranges (drained)
- 1/2 teaspoon vanilla extract
- 1 teaspoon sugar
- 1/2 cup plain fat-free yogurt
- 4 ounces fat-free cream cheese (room temperature)

Directions:

1. Put yogurt, cream cheese, vanilla, and sugar in a bowl. Mix using an electric mixer on high speed.

2. Put the drained fruits – pineapple, peaches, and oranges in another bowl. Toss until mixed. Fold in the cream cheese mixture. Cover the bowl with plastic and chill in the fridge.

3. Top with shredded coconut before serving.

Squash and Sweet Potato Pie

Serves: 8

Calories per serving: 210

Sodium per serving: 109 mg

Ingredients:

- 1/2 cup soy milk
- 1/2 cup silken tofu
- 1 buttercup squash (peeled, seeded, cooked_
- 1 sweet potato (peeled, cooked)
- 1 frozen pre-made 9-inch pie shell
- 3 tablespoons honey
- 1 teaspoon orange zest
- 1 teaspoon fresh grated ginger
- 1/2 teaspoon clove
- 1/2 teaspoon cinnamon

- 1/2 teaspoon nutmeg
- 1/2 teaspoon vanilla extract
- 1/4 cup rye flour
- 1/4 cup egg whites

Directions:

1. Put squash and sweet potato in a food processor. Process until pureed. Transfer to a bowl. Add the rest of the ingredients. Mix until combined.

2. Put pie shell on a baking sheet. Top with the mixture and bake in a preheated oven at 300 degrees F for 50 minutes.

Fruit Palette

Serves: 4

Calories per serving: 152

Sodium per serving: 3 mg

Ingredients:

- 1/2 cup powdered sugar
- 2 cups unsweetened frozen strawberries (thawed)
- 1/4 teaspoon sugar
- 1/4 teaspoon ground cinnamon
- Fresh mint leaves for garnish

- 1 kiwi (peeled and sliced)
- 1 plum (pitted and sliced)
- 1 pear (pitted and sliced)
- 1 peach (pitted and sliced)
- 1 star fruit (sliced)

Directions:

1. Mix to combine sugar and cinnamon in a small bowl.

2. Put powdered sugar and strawberries in a blender or food processor. Process until smooth. Divide into rimmed dessert plates. Top with sliced fruit and the sugar and cinnamon mixture.

3. Garnish with fresh mint before serving.

Very Berry Pie

Serves: 6

Calories per serving: 133

Sodium per serving: 169 mg

Ingredients:

- 6 mint leaves (for garnish)
- 6 tablespoons light whipped topping
- 6 single-serve graham cracker pie crusts
- 3/4 cup raspberries

- 3/4 cup sliced strawberries
- 1/2 cup fat-free, sugar-free instant vanilla pudding

Directions

1. Check package for directions on how to prepare the pudding. Divide among the pie crusts.

2. Mix raspberries and strawberries in a bowl. Put 2 tablespoons of the mixed berries on top of each pie and add a tablespoon of whipped topping.

3. Put mint leaves in each pie before serving.

Marinated Berries

Serves: 2

Calories per serving: 176

Sodium per serving: 56 mg

Ingredients:

- 2 shortbread biscuits
- 1/2 cup raspberries
- 1/2 cup blueberries
- 1/2 cup sliced strawberries
- 1 teaspoon vanilla extract
- 2 tablespoons brown sugar

- 1/4 cup balsamic vinegar

Directions:

1. Put vanilla, brown sugar, and vinegar in a bowl. Whisk until combined.

2. Toss to combine raspberries, blueberries, and strawberries in another bowl. Add the vinegar mixture and leave to marinate the fruits for 15 minutes.

3. Drain the liquid. Serve the berries along with shortbread biscuit.

Berry Apple Cobbler

Serves: 8

Calories per serving: 222

Sodium per serving: 202 mg

Ingredients:

- 12 ounces fresh or frozen blueberries
- 1 teaspoon ground cinnamon
- 2 tablespoons cornstarch
- 2 tablespoons sugar
- 1 tablespoon lemon juice
- 2 large apples, peeled, cored and thinly sliced

For the topping:

- 1 teaspoon vanilla extract
- 1/2 cup fat-free milk
- 4 tablespoons cold trans-free margarine (cubed)
- 1/4 teaspoon salt
- 1 1/2 teaspoons baking powder
- 2 tablespoons sugar
- 3/4 cup whole-wheat flour
- 3/4 cup all-purpose flour

Directions:

1. Put apple slices in a bowl. Add lemon juice and toss until coated.

2. Put cinnamon, cornstarch, and sugar in a small bowl. Add to the apple slices and gently toss until coated. Add the blueberries and gently mix until combined. Transfer to a lightly greased baking dish.

3. Put salt, baking powder, sugar, and flours in a bowl. Add cold margarine and cut using a fork until the mixture becomes similar to coarse crumbs. Add vanilla and milk. Mix until a dough forms.

4. Transfer dough to a lightly floured surface. Knead until smooth. Flatten into half an inch thickness using a rolling pin. Cut out shapes using a cookie cutter. Arrange the cut-outs on

top of the berry mixture. Bake in a preheated oven at 400 degrees F for 30 minutes.

Dipped Apples

Serves: 8

Calories per serving: 118

Sodium per serving: 202 mg

Ingredients:

- 1/2 cup orange juice
- 4 medium (cored and sliced)
- 2 tablespoons unsalted peanuts (chopped)
- 1 1/2 teaspoons vanilla
- 2 tablespoons brown sugar
- 8 ounces fat-free cream cheese (chilled)

Directions:

1. Prepare the dip. Leave cream cheese at room temperature for 5 minutes to soften. Place in a bowl along with vanilla and brown sugar. Mix well. Add chopped peanuts and mix until combined.

2. Put the apple slices in a bowl and coat with orange juice. Drain liquid and serve along with the dip.

Almond and Apricot Crisp

Serves: 6

Calories per serving: 134

Sodium per serving: 1 mg

Ingredients:

- 2 tablespoons honey
- 1 teaspoon anise seeds
- 1 tablespoon gluten-free oats
- 1/2 cup almonds (chopped)
- 1 pound apricots (halved, remove the pits, chopped)
- 1 teaspoon olive oil

Directions:

1. Arrange the chopped apricots in a glass pie dish. Add anise seeds, oats, and almonds. Scoop honey on top. Bake in a preheated oven at 350 degrees F for 25 minutes.

Spiced Carrot Quick Bread

Serves: 17

Calories per serving: 110

Sodium per serving: 82 mg

Ingredients:

- 1/2 teaspoon baking soda
- 2 teaspoons baking powder
- 1 cup whole-wheat flour
- 1/2 cup all-purpose flour (sifted)
- 1/4 teaspoon ground ginger
- 1/2 teaspoon ground cinnamon
- 1 tablespoon finely chopped walnuts
- 2 tablespoons golden raisins
- 1 1/2 cups shredded carrots
- 1 teaspoon grated orange rind
- 1 teaspoon vanilla extract
- 2 egg whites (beaten)
- 2 tablespoons unsweetened orange juice
- 1/3 cup skim milk
- 1/4 cup, plus 2 tablespoons firmly packed brown sugar
- 1/3 cup trans fat-free margarine (room temperature)

Directions:

1. Put ground ginger, ground cinnamon, baking soda, baking powder, and flours in a bowl. Mix until combined.

2. Put sugar and margarine in another bowl. Mix well. Add orange rind, vanilla, egg, orange juice, and milk. Mix well. Stir in walnuts,

raisins, and carrots. Add the flour mixture and mix until combined.

3. Transfer batter to a lightly greased loaf pan. Bake in a preheated oven at 375 degrees F for 45 minutes.

Poached Pears

Serves: 4

Calories per serving: 140

Sodium per serving: 9 mg

Ingredients:

- 2 tablespoons orange zest
- 1/2 cup fresh raspberries
- 4 whole pears (peeled, cored)
- 1 teaspoon ground nutmeg
- 1 teaspoon ground cinnamon
- 1/4 cup apple juice
- 1 cup orange juice

Directions:

1. Put nutmeg, cinnamon, and the juices in a small bowl. Mix well.

2. Transfer the juice mixture in a shallow pan over medium flame. Add the pears and simmer

for half an hour while stirring often. Turn off heat before the liquid boils.

3. Place pears in serving plates and garnish with orange zest and raspberries.

Cheesecake with Lemon

Serves: 8

Calories per serving: 80

Sodium per serving: 252 mg

Ingredients:

- Lemon zest
- 2 cups low-fat cottage cheese
- 1 teaspoon vanilla
- 1/4 cup sugar
- Egg substitute equivalent to 2 egg whites or 1 egg
- 1/2 cup skim milk (heated through)
- 2 tablespoons lemon juice
- 1 envelope unflavored gelatin
- 2 tablespoons cold water

Directions:

1. Put lemon juice, gelatin, and water in a blender. Process for 2 minutes. Add hot milk and process until the gelatin is dissolved. Add

cheese, vanilla, sugar, and egg substitute. Blend until smooth. Transfer to a flat dish and keep in the fridge for 3 hours.

2. Garnish with grated lemon zest before serving.

Creamy Berry

Serves: 6

Calories per serving: 136

Sodium per serving: 95 mg

Ingredients:

- 1 quart fresh strawberries, hulled and halved, reserve whole 6 pieces as garnishing)
- 2 tablespoons amaretto liqueur
- 1/2 cup brown sugar
- 1 1/2 cups fat-free sour cream

Directions:

1. Whisk liqueur, brown sugar, and sour cream in a bowl until combined. Transfer to a large bowl and add the halved berries. Toss until coated. Cover the bowl and chill in the fridge for an hour.

2. Top each serving with whole strawberries.

Berry Crepes

Serves: 4

Calories per serving: 143

Sodium per serving: 161 mg

Ingredients:

- 2 tablespoons caramel sauce (warmed)
- 1 teaspoon powdered sugar for garnishing
- 8 strawberries (hulled and sliced)
- 2 prepackaged crepes
- 2 teaspoons vanilla extract
- 2 tablespoons powdered sugar (sifted)
- 4 tablespoons cream cheese (room temperature)

Directions:

1. Whisk cream cheese in a bowl until smooth. Add vanilla and powdered sugar as you whisk. Mix until combined.

2. Scoop half of the mixture on each crepe and spread evenly. Add 2 tablespoons strawberries on top. Roll them up and arrange on a lightly

greased baking dish. Bake in a preheated oven at 325 degrees F for 10 minutes.

3. Cut each crepe in half. Serve each piece with half a tablespoons caramel sauce and a sprinkle of powdered sugar.

Strawberry Sorbet

Serves: 6

Calories per serving: 62

Sodium per serving: 1 mg

Ingredients:

- 1 tablespoon dark honey
- 4 cups strawberries (hulled and halved)
- 4 strawberries (coarsely chopped)
- 3/4 cup balsamic vinegar

Directions:

1. Simmer vinegar in a saucepan over medium-low flame until reduced by half. Turn off heat and leave to cool.

2. Process the berries in a food processor or blender until smooth. Sieve as you press the

solids using the back of a spoon. Collect all juice in a bowl. Add honey and vinegar. Mix well. Cover the bowl and keep in the fridge for a couple of hours.

3. Transfer the mixture to an ice cream maker. Process according to the indicated directions in the package. Freeze until ready to serve. This will last up to 2 days. Top with chopped berries before serving.

Peach Crumble

Serves: 8

Calories per serving: 152

Sodium per serving: 41 mg

Ingredients:

- 1/3 teaspoon ground cinnamon
- Juice from 1 lemon
- 8 ripe peaches (peeled, pitted and sliced)
- 1/4 cup quick-cooking oats (uncooked)
- 2 tablespoons trans-free margarine (thinly sliced)
- 1/4 cup packed dark brown sugar
- 1/2 cup whole-wheat flour
- 1/4 teaspoon ground nutmeg

Directions:

1. Place the pie slices in a lightly greased pie plate. Sprinkle with nutmeg, cinnamon, and lemon juice.

2. Put brown sugar and flour in a bowl. Mix well. Add margarine. Crumble using your fingers as you mix it with the sugar mixture. Add oats and mix well. Spread on top of the peaches.

3. Bake in a preheated oven at 375 degrees F for half an hour. Slice into 8 and serve.

Strawberry Shortcake

Serves: 8

Calories per serving: 218

Sodium per serving: 75 mg

Ingredients:

For the shortcake:

- 3/4 cup fat-free milk (chilled)
- 1/4 cup trans-free margarine (chilled)
- 1 tablespoon sugar

- 2 1/2 teaspoons low-sodium baking powder
- 1/4 cup all-purpose flour (sifted)
- 1 3/4 cups whole-wheat pastry flour (sifted)

For the topping:

- 3/4 cup vanilla or plain fat-free yogurt
- 6 cups fresh strawberries (hulled and sliced)

Directions:

1. Sift to combine sugar, baking powder, and flours. Add the chilled margarine and cut using a fork until the mixture becomes similar to coarse crumbs. Stir in chilled milk and mix until moist.

2. Transfer dough to a floured surface. Knead until smooth. Flatten into 1/4-inch thickness and cut into 8 squares. Arrange on a lightly greased baking sheet. Bake in a preheated oven at 425 degrees F for 12 minutes.

3. Top each biscuit with 1 1/2 tablespoons of yogurt and 3/4 cup strawberries.

Very Chocolate Cake

Serves: 18

Calories per serving: 183

Sodium per serving: 220 mg

Ingredients:

- 2 cups boiling water
- 1/2 cup canola oil
- 2 tablespoons vinegar
- 1 tablespoon vanilla
- 2 1/4 teaspoons baking soda
- 1/2 teaspoon salt
- 3 tablespoons unsweetened cocoa powder
- 1 cup sugar
- 3 cups whole-wheat pastry flour

Directions:

1. Put baking soda, salt, cocoa powder, sugar, and flour in a baking pan. Whisk until combined. Make 3 holes using a spoon. Put oil in the first hole, vinegar in another and vanilla in the last hole. Gradually add boiling water as you whisk. Mix for a couple of minutes until combined.

2. Bake in a preheated oven at 350 degrees F for 30 minutes. Allow to cool before dividing into 18.

Nutty Bar with Fruits

Serves: 24

Calories per serving: 70

Sodium per serving: 4 mg

Ingredients:

- 2 tablespoons cornstarch
- 1/4 cup chopped dried pineapple
- 1/4 cup honey
- 1/4 cup chopped dried figs
- 1/4 cup chopped dried apricots
- 1/4 cup chopped almonds
- 1/4 cup wheat germ
- 1/4 cup flaxseed flour
- 1/2 cup oats
- 1/2 cup quinoa flour

Directions:

1. Put all ingredients in a bowl and mix until combined. Transfer to a pan lined with parchment paper. Press to compress into 1/2-inch thickness. Bake for 20 minutes at 300 degrees F. Leave to cool before cutting into squares.

Fruity Compote ala Mode

Serves: 8

Calories per serving: 228

Sodium per serving: 70 mg

Ingredients:

- 4 cups fat-free vanilla frozen yogurt
- 1/4 teaspoon ground ginger
- 1/4 teaspoon ground nutmeg
- 1 teaspoon ground cinnamon
- 1 12-ounce package mixed dried fruit
- 1/2 cup orange juice
- 1 1/4 cups water

Directions:

1. Put water in a saucepan over medium flame. Stir as you add ginger, nutmeg, cinnamon, dried fruit, and orange juice. Cover and simmer for 10 minutes. Stir and turn heat to low. Simmer for 10 more minutes.

2. Serve cold or warm along with frozen yogurt.

Coffee Cake with Crumbs

Serves: 10

Calories per serving: 281

Sodium per serving: 198 mg

Ingredients:

For the topping:

2 tablespoons trans-free margarine, melted

1/4 cup chopped pecans

1/2 cup packed brown sugar

1/4 cup whole-wheat flour

For the cake:

- 8 ounces fat-free sour cream
- 1 1/4 teaspoons vanilla
- 1/4 teaspoon baking soda
- 1 1/2 teaspoons baking powder
- 3/4 cup sugar
- 3/4 cup whole-wheat flour
- 3/4 cup all-purpose flour
- 1/2 cup chopped dried fruits
- 1 cup chopped fresh cranberries
- 4 tablespoons trans-free margarine
- 2 egg whites

Directions:

1. Prepare the topping. Put chopped pecans, brown sugar, and flour in a bowl. Mix well. Add melted margarine and mix until crumbly.

2. Put flour, baking soda, baking powder, and sugar in another bowl. Whisk until combined.

3. In another bowl, put margarine, egg whites, sour cream, and vanilla. Beat using an electric mixer on low speed. Gradually add the sour cream mixture. Mix until smooth.

4. Scoop half of the batter to the pan. Add chopped fruit and top with the rest of the batter. Add topping and bake in a preheated oven at 350 degrees F for 45 minutes.

5. Slice and serve.

Cookies and Cream Shake

Serves: 3

Calories per serving: 270

Sodium per serving: 224 mg

Ingredients:

- 6 chocolate wafer cookies (crushed)
- 3 cups fat-free vanilla ice cream
- 1 1/3 cups vanilla soy milk (chilled)

Directions:

1. Put ice cream and soy milk in a blender. Process until frothy. Add cookies and pulse up to 6 times. Transfer to serving glasses and serve t once.

Fruitcake

Serves: 12

Calories per serving: 229

Sodium per serving: 117 mg

Ingredients:

- Zest and juice of 1 lemon
- Zest and juice of 1 medium orange
- 1/2 cup walnuts (crushed or chopped)
- 1 egg
- 1/2 teaspoon baking powder
- 1/2 teaspoon baking soda
- 1 cup whole-wheat pastry flour
- 1/4 cup flaxseed flour
- 1/2 cup rolled oats
- 1/4 cup sugar
- 2 tablespoons real vanilla extract
- 1/2 cup unsweetened apple juice
- 1/2 cup crushed pineapple packed in juice (drained)
- 1/2 cup unsweetened applesauce
- 2 cups assorted chopped dried fruits

Directions:

1. Put vanilla, fruit juices and zests, pineapple, applesauce, and dried fruit in a bowl. Toss until combined. Let stand for 20 minutes.

2. Whisk baking powder, baking soda, flours, oats, and sugar in a bowl until combined. Add the fruit mixture and mix well. Add walnuts and egg. Mix until combined.

3. Transfer mixture to a loaf pan lined with parchment paper. Bake for an hour at 325 degrees F. Allow to cool for 30 minutes before unmolding.

Apple Dumplings

Serves: 8

Calories per serving: 178

Sodium per serving: 14 mg

Ingredients:

For the dough:

- 2 tablespoons brandy or apple liquor
- 2 tablespoons rolled oats
- 2 tablespoons buckwheat flour
- 1 cup whole-wheat flour
- 1 teaspoon honey
- 1 tablespoon butter

For the apple filling:

- Zest of one lemon
- 2 tablespoons honey
- 1 teaspoon nutmeg
- 6 large tart apples, thinly sliced

Directions:

1. Put oats, flours, honey, and butter in a food processor. Process until combined and the mixture looks like a fine meal. Add liquor and pulse three or four times. Transfer to a plastic, wrap around the mixture and leave in the fridge for 2 hours.

2. Mix honey, nutmeg, lemon zest, and apples in a bowl.

3. Transfer cold dough to a floured surface. Roll into 1/4-inch thickness and cut into circles using a muffin tin. Place each circle in a greased muffin tin. Gently push the dough, add apple mixture, fold the sides and pinch the top part until sealed.

4. Bake in a preheated oven at 350 degrees F for 30 minutes.

Rice Pudding with Fruits

Serves: 8

Calories per serving: 257

Sodium per serving: 193 mg

Ingredients:

- 6 egg whites
- 1 teaspoon vanilla extract
- 1/2 teaspoon lemon zest
- 1/2 cup brown sugar
- 4 cups evaporated fat-free milk
- 1 cup long-grain brown rice
- 2 cups water
- 1/4 cup dried apricots (chopped)
- 1/4 cup raisins
- 1/4 cup crushed pineapple

Directions:

1. Pour 2 cups of water in a saucepan over medium-high flame. Bring to a boil. Add rice and cook for 10 minutes. Drain cooking liquid.

2. Put brown sugar and evaporated milk in the same pan. Stir until heated through. Add vanilla extract, lemon zest, and the cooked rice. Turn heat to low and simmer for half an hour. Turn off the heat and leave to cool.

3. Whisk egg whites in a bowl. Pour on top of the rice mixture. Add apricots, raisins, and pineapple. Mix well.

4. Transfer mixture to a lightly greased baking dish. Bake in a preheated oven at 325 degrees F for 20 minutes.

Sliced Orange with Syrup

Serves: 4

Calories per serving: 183

Sodium per serving: 3 mg

Ingredients:

- Zest of 1 orange (cut into thin strips)
- 4 oranges

For syrup:

- 2 tablespoons dark honey
- 1 1/2 cups fresh orange juice (strained)

For garnishing:

- 4 fresh mint sprigs
- 2 tablespoons orange liqueur (optional)

Directions:

1. Cut a thin slice off the bottom and top parts of each orange. Stand upright, peel and remove membrane and white pith. Cut into half an inch thick slices and place on a dish. Repeat the process until you're done with all the oranges.

2. Put water and strips of zest in a saucepan over medium-high flame. Bring to a boil. Drain and soak the zest in cold water.

3. Prepare the syrup. Put honey and orange juice in a pan over medium-high flame. Bring to a boil while constantly stirring. Turn heat to low and simmer for 5 minutes. Remove orange zest from water and add to the pan. Cook for 5 more minutes as you stir.

4. Pour syrup on top of the oranges. Cover with plastic and chill in the fridge for 3 hours.

5. Scoop 1 1/2 teaspoons of orange liqueur in each serving and top with mint.

Blackberry Iced Tea

Serves: 6

Calories per serving: 25

Sodium per serving: 3 mg

Ingredients:

- Crushed ice cubes
- Sugar substitute to taste
- 1 cup unsweetened cranberry juice

- 1 tablespoon minced fresh ginger
- 8 3-inch-long cinnamon sticks
- 12 blackberry herbal tea bags
- 6 cups water

Directions:

1. Put water in a saucepan over medium-high flame. Add ginger, 2 cinnamon sticks, and tea bags before the water boils. Turn off the heat and cover the pan. Leave to steep for 15 minutes.

2. Sift mixture and pour in a pitcher, Add sweetener and juice. Put in the fridge for a couple of hours.

3. Place crushed ice in each serving glass. Pour the tea and top with cinnamon sticks.

Hurricane Punch

Serves: 6

Calories per serving: 64

Sodium per serving: 6 mg

Ingredients:

1 cup ice, plus more for serving

8 ounces cranberry juice

Juice of 1 lemon

2 cups citrus fruit

1 1/2 cups chopped pineapple

Directions:

1. Puree all ingredients, except ice, in a blender. Add a cup of ice and process until combined. Transfer to serving glasses, add ice and top with orange slices or pineapple chunks.

Island Chiller

Serves: 16

Calories per serving: 72

Sodium per serving: 7 mg

Ingredients:

- 3 cups orange juice
- 2 quarts carbonated water (chilled)
- 16 fresh strawberries
- 2 10-ounce packages frozen unsweetened strawberries
- 1 1/2 cans crushed pineapple with juice

Directions:

1. Put orange juice, pineapple and juice, and frozen strawberries in a blender. Process until smooth. Transfer to ice cube trays and freeze.

2. Pour half a cup of carbonated water to each serving glass and add 3 strawberry cubes. Top with fresh berry and serve.

Fruity Smoothie

Serves: 4

Calories per serving: 72

Sodium per serving: 7 mg

Ingredients:

- 1 tablespoon honey
- 1 cup cold water
- Juice of 2 oranges
- 1 cup fresh strawberries (remove stems)
- 1/2 cup cantaloupe or other melon chunks
- 1 cup fresh pineapple chunks

Directions:

1. Discard rind of melon and pineapple and slice them into chunks. Place in a blender, add the rest of the ingredients and process until smooth.

Champagne Cider

Serves: 4

Calories per serving: 55

Sodium per serving: 4 mg

Ingredients:

- 2 cups lemon-flavored sparkling water
- 1 1/2 teaspoons fresh lemon juice
- 2 cups unsweetened apple juice or apple cider

Directions:

1. Chill wine or champagne glass. Pour sparkling water, lemon juice, and apple juice. Stir and serve.

Cranberry Spritzer

Serves: 10

Calories per serving: 100

Sodium per serving: 9 mg

Ingredients:

- 10 lemon or lime wedges

- 1 cup raspberry sherbet
- 1/4 cup sugar
- 1 quart seltzer water
- 1/2 cup fresh lemon juice
- 1 quart reduced-calorie cranberry juice

Directions:

1. Mix carbonated water, lemon juice, and carbonated juice in a pitcher. Keep in the fridge for an hour. Add sherbet and sugar. Pour into chilled serving glasses and top with lime or lemon wedges.

Lavender Lemonade

Serves: 16

Calories per serving: 33

Sodium per serving: 7 mg

Ingredients:

- Cold water
- 2 tablespoons Splenda sweetener
- 1 cup lemon juice
- 1 tablespoon dried lavender flowers
- 1/4 cup granulated sugar
- 1 16-ounce package blueberries
- 2 cups water

Directions:

1. Put 4 cups of ice in a pitcher.

2. Pour 2 cups of water in a saucepan over medium-high flame. Bring to a boil. Add lavender, sugar, and blueberries. Boil until the sugar dissolves or about 5 minutes. Strain and pour liquid on the pitcher of ice. Add Splenda and lemon juice. Fill pitcher with cold water and mix until combined.

Iced Latte

Serves: 4

Calories per serving: 70

Sodium per serving: 69 mg

Ingredients:

- 1 teaspoon ground espresso beans
- 1 cup fat-free whipped topping
- Ice cubes
- 2 tablespoons sugar-free almond syrup
- 1 1/2 cups fat-free milk
- 2 tablespoons golden brown sugar
- 2 cups brewed decaffeinated espresso coffee (cooled)

Directions:

1. Put syrup, milk, brown sugar, and espresso in a pitcher. Mix well. Put in the fridge for an hour.

2. Put ice cubes in serving glasses. Pour coffee and top each glass with 1/4 cup of the whipped topping and espresso beans.

Orange Smoothie

Serves: 4

Calories per serving: 101

Sodium per serving: 40 mg

Ingredients:

- 4 peeled orange segments
- 5 ice cubes
- 1/2 teaspoon vanilla extract
- 1 teaspoon grated orange zest
- 1 tablespoon dark honey
- 1/3 cup silken or soft tofu
- 1 cup light vanilla soy milk (chilled)
- 1 1/2 cups orange juice (chilled)

Directions:

1. Put ice cubes in a blender. Add vanilla, orange zest, honey, tofu, soy milk, and orange juice. Blend until smooth. Transfer to serving

glasses and top each serving with an orange segment.

Green Smoothie

Serves: 4

Calories per serving: 64

Sodium per serving: 15 mg

Ingredients:

- 1 cup cold water (or ice)
- Fresh mint to taste
- 2 ounces fresh raw baby spinach
- 1/2 cup other berries, such as blueberries or blackberries
- 1/2 cup strawberries
- Juice of 1 lemon 1 banana

Directions:

1. Puree all ingredients in a juicer or blender. Transfer to serving glasses and serve.

Cranberry and Watermelon Drink

Serves: 6

Calories per serving: 84

Sodium per serving: 9 mg

Ingredients:

1 lime (sliced into 6)

1/4 cup fresh lime juice

1 cup fruit-sweetened cranberry juice

2 1/2 pounds seedless watermelon, rind removed and diced

Directions:

1. Puree melon in a food processor or blender. Sift and transfer juice to a pitcher. Add lime juice and cranberry juice. Mix well. Keep in the fridge for an hour.

2. Transfer to serving glasses and top with lime slices.

Chapter 7 – Recipes for Snacks and Side Dish

Fish Tacos

Serves: 6

Calories per serving (2 tacos): 284

Sodium per serving: 278 mg

Ingredients:

- 2 medium limes (cut into wedges)
- 1 cup chopped fresh cilantro
- 2 cups red cabbage (chopped)
- 12 corn tortillas
- 6 mahi-mahi fillets
- Hot pepper sauce
- Salsa verde (optional)
- 1 teaspoon pepper
- 1 teaspoon salt
- 1 teaspoon paprika
- 1 teaspoon ground cardamom
- 1/4 cup olive oil

Directions:

1. Put olive oil, paprika, ground cardamom, salt, and pepper in a bowl. Mix until combined.

2. Arrange fillets on a baking dish. Cover with the seasoning mixture. Cover and leave in the fridge for 30 minutes.

3. Drain liquid from the fillets. Place on an oiled grill rack over medium-high heat. Cover and grill for 5 minutes. Transfer to a plate. Warm the tortillas on the grill for 45 seconds.

4. Put fish inside each tortilla. Add cilantro and red cabbage. Squeeze a bit of hot pepper sauce and lime juice. You can also add salsa verde if preferred. Fold the sides of the tortilla. Add more pepper sauce, if you want and serve with lime wedges.

Corn Pudding

Serves: 8

Calories per serving: 213

Sodium per serving: 44 mg

Ingredients:

- 1/2 cup raisins
- 1/8 teaspoon ginger
- 1/8 teaspoon clove
- 1/8 teaspoon nutmeg
- 1/4 teaspoon cinnamon
- 1/4 cup maple syrup
- 2 cups coarse cornmeal

- 3 cups skim milk
- 3 cups water

Directions:

1. Put milk and water in a saucepan over medium-high flame. Bring to a boil. Add cornmeal. Mix to free it from lumps. Bring to another boil. Turn heat to low, cover and simmer for 15 minutes while occasionally stirring.

2. Remove pan from the stove. Add the rest of the ingredients. Mix well and leave for 15 minutes.

Mashed Cauliflower

Serves: 4

Calories per serving: 67

Sodium per serving: 60 mg

Ingredients:

- 1 tablespoon non-hydrogenated soft-tub margarine
- 1 leek (white part, cut into 4)
- Pepper to taste
- 1 garlic clove
- 1 head cauliflower

Directions:

1. Cut cauliflower into florets. Steam along with leeks and garlic for 30 minutes. Transfer to a food processor. Process until the consistency is similar to mashed potatoes.

2. Add pepper and margarine before serving.

Braised Kale

Serves: 6

Calories per serving: 70

Sodium per serving: 133 mg

Ingredients:

- 1/8 teaspoon freshly ground black pepper
- 1/4 teaspoon salt
- 1 tablespoon fresh lemon juice
- 1 cup cherry tomatoes (halved)
- 1/2 cup low-sodium vegetable stock (or broth)
- 1 pound kale (remove tough stems and coarsely chop the leaves)
- 4 garlic cloves (thinly sliced)
- 2 teaspoons extra-virgin olive oil

Directions:

1. Heat oil in a pan over medium flame. Add garlic and cook for a minute or until lightly golden. Add stock and kale. Cover the pan and turn heat to medium-low. Cook for 5 minutes.

2. Remove the cover and add tomatoes. Continue cooking for 7 minutes. Turn off the heat and stir in pepper, salt, and lemon juice.

Grilled Shrimp with Lime Kabob

Serves: 4

Calories per serving: 167

Sodium per serving: 284 mg

Ingredients:

- 1/4 teaspoon pepper
- 1/4 teaspoon ground cumin
- 1/4 teaspoon salt
- 3 garlic cloves (minced)
- 2 tablespoons olive oil
- 1 jalapeno pepper (seeded and minced)
- 1/3 cup lime juice
- 1 1/2 teaspoons grated lime zest
- 1/3 cup chopped fresh cilantro
- Lime slices
- 1 pound uncooked shrimp (peeled and deveined)

Directions:

1. Put shrimp in a bowl. Add the rest of the ingredients, except the lime slices, and toss until combined. Leave for 15 minutes.

2. Thread lime slices and seasoned shrimp on 4 metal skewers. Put on a grill rack over medium heat. Cover and grill each side for 4 minutes.

Tasty Turkey Burgers

Serves: 4

Calories per serving: 315

Sodium per serving: 482 mg

Ingredients:

- 4 whole wheat hamburger buns (split)
- 1 pound lean ground turkey
- 1/8 teaspoon pepper
- 1/4 teaspoon garlic salt
- 1 garlic clove (minced)
- 2 tablespoons quick-cooking oats
- 3 tablespoons barbecue sauce (mesquite smoke-flavored)
- 1/4 cup freshly chopped basil

Directions:

1. Put pepper, garlic salt, oats, barbecue sauce, and basil in a bowl. Mix well. Add turkey and gently mix until combined. Divide mixture into 4 and shape each into a patty with 1/2-inch thickness.

2. Place patties on a greased grill rack over medium heat. Cover and grill each side for 7 minutes. Slice and grill the buns for 30 seconds. Put the burgers in the buns and add your preferred toppings.

Mediterranean Hummus Dip

Serves: 12

Calories per serving: 88

Sodium per serving: 275 mg

Ingredients:

- Baked pita chips
- 1 cup crumbled feta cheese
- 1 large English cucumber (chopped)
- 2 medium tomatoes (seeded and chopped)
- 1/2 cup Greek olives (chopped)
- 1/4 cup red onion (finely chopped)
- 1 10-ounce carton hummus

Directions:

1. Put hummus in a round dish. Spread all over. Add cheese, cucumber, tomatoes, olives, and onion. Keep in the fridge until ready to serve. You can use this as dipping for crackers, sliced veggies or chips.

Tuna Kabobs

Serves: 4

Calories per serving: 205

Sodium per serving: 50 mg

Ingredients:

- 1 medium mango (peeled and cubed)
- 2 large sweet red peppers (chopped)
- 1 teaspoon pepper (coarsely ground)
- 1 pound tuna steaks (cut into 1-inch cubes)
- 2 tablespoons lime juice
- 2 tablespoons fresh parsley (coarsely chopped)
- 1 jalapeno pepper (seeded and chopped)
- 4 green onions (chopped)
- 1/2 cup frozen corn (thawed)

Directions:

1. Prepare the salsa. Put corn, lime juice, parsley, jalapeno, and onions in a bowl. Mix until combined. Set aside.

2. Season tuna with pepper. Thread mango, tuna, and red peppers in an alternate fashion on 4 metal skewers. Put on a lightly greased grill rack over medium heat. Cover and grill for 12 minutes.

3. Serve kabobs along with the prepared salsa.

Tasty Zucchini

Serves: 4

Calories per serving: 64

Sodium per serving: 9 mg

Ingredients:

- 2 tablespoons lemon juice
- 2 scallions (chopped)
- 2 tablespoons fresh cilantro
- 1 teaspoon dill weed
- 2 cups thinly sliced green zucchini
- 2 cups thinly sliced yellow zucchini
- 1 tablespoon olive oil

Directions:

1. Heat oil in a pan over medium flame. Add zucchini and cook for 5 minutes while constantly stirring. Stir in scallions, cilantro, and dill. Transfer to a bowl.

2. Add lemon juice before serving.

Root Veggies with Glaze

Serves: 4

Calories per serving: 57

Sodium per serving: 24 mg

Ingredients:

- 1/2 cup carrots (cut into 1-inch pieces)
- 1/2 cup onions (cut into 1-inch pieces)
- 1 1/2 cups water
- 1 teaspoon olive oil
- 2 teaspoons sugar
- 1/2 cup new potatoes (cubed)
- 1/2 cup turnips (chopped)

Directions:

1. Put water in a pan over medium flame. Add potatoes, turnips, carrots, and onions. Simmer for 15 minutes. Drain cooking liquid and add olive oil and a sprinkle of sugar. Turn heat to medium-high, stir the veggies and cook until golden.

Lemon Rice

Serves: 8

Calories per serving: 201

Sodium per serving: 44 mg

Ingredients:

- 2 teaspoons lemon zest
- 3 tablespoons lemon juice
- 1 3/4 cup unsalted chicken broth
- 1 cup uncooked brown rice
- 1/2 cup slivered almonds (coarsely chopped)
- 1 tablespoon trans-free margarine
- 1/4 teaspoon ground nutmeg
- 1/2 teaspoon ground cinnamon
- 1/4 cup chopped onions
- 2 tablespoons honey
- 1/2 cup frozen peas
- 1/2 cup golden raisins
- 1/3 cup water

Directions:

1. Put almonds in a baking tray. Bake in a preheated oven at 325 degrees F for 10 minutes while stirring every 2 minutes. Leave to cool.

2. Heat broth in a saucepan over medium flame. Add margarine, nutmeg, cinnamon, onion, lemon zest and juice, and rice. Mix well. Cover the pan and simmer for 30 minutes while occasionally stirring.

3. Put raisins and water in a saucepan over medium flame. Cover and simmer for 5 minutes. Stir in the pea and simmer for a minute. Add mixture to the rice. Simmer for 20 more minutes.

4. Fluff the cooked rice and transfer to a bowl. Add honey and toasted almonds on top.

Asian Asparagus Dish

Serves: 6

Calories per serving: 24

Sodium per serving: 26 mg

Ingredients:

- 1 1/2 pounds fresh asparagus (ends removed and cut into strips)
- 1 teaspoon reduced-sodium soy sauce
- 1/2 teaspoon sugar

- 1/2 cup water

Directions:

1. Heat soy sauce, sugar, and water in a pan over high flame. Bring to a boil. Stir in asparagus and turn heat to low. Simmer for 4 minutes.

Roasted Bananas and Potatoes

Serves: 6

Calories per serving: 156

Sodium per serving: 64 mg

Ingredients:

- 3 tablespoons brown sugar
- 1/4 teaspoon ground nutmeg
- 1/4 teaspoon ground cardamom
- 1/2 teaspoon ground cinnamon
- Chopped parsley for garnish
- Red pepper flakes to taste
- 2 tablespoons orange juice
- 2 medium bananas (peeled and halved)
- 1 1/2 pounds sweet potatoes (rinsed)

Directions:

1. Poke sweet potatoes using a fork to create several holes. Place in a greased baking dish and bake in a preheated oven at 375 degrees F for an hour. Leave to cool before removing the peel.

2. Arrange the banana halves in the greased baking dish. Bake for 15 minutes. Transfer to a bowl. Add orange juice and mash the bananas as you mix. Add brown sugar, spices, and sweet potatoes. Blend using an electric mixer until smooth. Transfer to a heatproof bowl. Bake until warmed.

3. Top with chopped parsley before serving.

Broccoli with Lemon and Garlic

Serves: 4

Calories per serving: 45

Sodium per serving: 153 mg

Ingredients:

- 1/4 teaspoon ground black pepper
- 1/4 teaspoon kosher salt
- 1 teaspoon lemon zest
- 1 tablespoon minced garlic
- 1 teaspoon olive oil
- 4 cups broccoli florets

Directions:

1. Pour a cup of water in a saucepan over medium-high flame. Bring to a boil. Add the broccoli and cook until tender. This will take about 3 minutes. Drain water.

2. Heat oil in a pan over medium-high flame. Add garlic and cook for 30 seconds while stirring. Add pepper, salt, lemon zest, and broccoli. Transfer to a serving platter and serve.

Braised Celery Root

Serves: 6

Calories per serving: 54

Sodium per serving: 206 mg

Ingredients:

- 2 teaspoons fresh thyme leaves
- 1/4 teaspoon freshly ground black pepper
- 1/4 teaspoon salt
- 1 teaspoon Dijon mustard
- 1/4 cup sour cream
- 1 celery root (peeled and diced)
- 1 cup vegetable stock (or broth)

Directions:

1. Pour stock in a pan over high flame. Bring to a boil. Add celery root. Turn heat to low and cover the pan. Simmer for 12 minutes while occasionally stirring. Scoop out celery root to a bowl. Loosely cover with foil to keep warm.

2. Turn heat of the stove to high and bring the cooking liquid to a boil. Remove from heat. Add pepper, salt, mustard, and sour cream. Whisk until combined. Turn on heat to medium. Add thyme and celery root. Cook until warmed.

Brown Rice Pilaf

Serves: 8

Calories per serving: 153

Sodium per serving: 222 mg

Ingredients:

- 1/4 teaspoon saffron threads or ground turmeric
- 3/4 teaspoon salt (divided)
- 2 cups water
- 1 1/8 cups dark brown rice (rinsed and drained)
- 1/4 cup dried apricots (chopped)
- 1/4 cup chopped pistachio nuts

- 1 1/2 tablespoons pistachio oil or canola oil
- 3 tablespoons fresh orange juice
- 1/2 teaspoon grated orange zest

Directions:

1. Put water, saffron, 1/4 teaspoon of salt, and rice in a saucepan over high flame. Bring to a boil. Turn heat to low and cover the pan. Simmer for 45 minutes. Transfer to a bowl and loosely cover with foil to keep warm.

2. Put the rest of the salt, oil, and orange zest and juice in a bowl. Whisk until combined. Pour over the rice. Add apricots and nuts. Toss until coated.

Black Bean Cakes

Serves: 8

Calories per serving: 196

Sodium per serving: 156 mg

Ingredients:

- 2 tablespoons olive oil
- 1/2 teaspoon salt
- 1/2 cup chopped fresh cilantro
- 8 garlic cloves (chopped)

- 4 cups water
- 2 cups dried black beans (picked over, washed, soaked overnight, and drained)

Directions:

1. Put water and black beans in a pan over high flame. Bring to a boil. Turn heat to low and simmer for 70 minutes while partially covered. Drain the liquid.

2. Put garlic and beans in a bowl. Mash as you mix. Add salt and cilantro. Mix well. Use your hands to form 8 cakes from the mixture. Arrange on a plate and keep in the fridge for an hour.

3. Heat oil in a pan over medium flame. Cook the cakes for 5 minutes or until crisp.

4. Serve at once.

Baby Carrots with Mint

Serves: 6

Calories per serving: 44

Sodium per serving: 51 mg

Ingredients:

- 1/8 teaspoon ground cinnamon

- 1/2 tablespoon fresh mint leaves (chopped)
- 1 tablespoon cornstarch
- 1/4 cup apple juice (100 percent)
- 1 pound baby carrots (rinsed)
- 6 cups water

Directions:

1. Heat water in a pan over medium-high flame. Add carrots and cook for 10 minutes. Drain and transfer carrots to a bowl.

2. Put cornstarch and apple juice in a pan over medium flame. Stir for 5 minutes or until thick. Add cinnamon and mint.

3. Serve carrots along with sauce.

Mushroom and Brown Rice Pilaf

Serves: 6

Calories per serving: 180

Sodium per serving: 25 mg

Ingredients:

- 1/2 cup fresh parsley (chopped)
- 2 tablespoons Swiss cheese (finely grated)
- 1/2 pound asparagus tips

- 1/8 teaspoon ground nutmeg
- 1/2 pound fresh mushrooms (thinly sliced)
- 1 small onion (chopped)
- 1 teaspoon low-sodium chicken-flavored bouillon granules
- 3 cups water
- 1 cup brown rice
- 1 tablespoon olive oil

Directions:

1. Heat oil in a pan over medium flame. Add rice and cook until toasted. Add water, nutmeg, mushrooms, onion, and bouillon granules. Bring to a boil. Turn heat to low and cover the pan. Simmer for half an hour. Add water if you need to.

2. Chop off the woody stems of the asparagus and cut into small pieces. Add to the rice mixture and cover the pan. Cook for 5 minutes.

3. Add parsley and grated cheese before serving.

Hazelnut Gremolata with Asparagus

Serves: 4

Calories per serving: 50

Sodium per serving: 148 mg

Ingredients:

- 1/4 teaspoon salt
- 1 teaspoon extra-virgin olive oil
- 2 teaspoons fresh lemon juice
- 1/4 teaspoon finely grated lemon zest, plus extra for garnish
- 1 tablespoon finely chopped toasted hazelnuts
- 1 tablespoon chopped fresh flat-leaf parsley, plus sprigs for garnish
- 1 garlic clove (minced)
- 1 pound asparagus (peeled if skin is thick, tough ends removed)

Directions:

1. Steam asparagus for 4 minutes or until tender-crisp. Transfer to a bowl. Add salt, olive oil, lemon juice, 1/4 teaspoon lemon zest, hazelnuts, chopped parsley, and garlic. Toss until coated.

2. Transfer to a plate and garnish with lemon zest and parsley sprigs before serving.

Shallots and Brussel Sprouts

Serves: 4

Calories per serving: 104

Sodium per serving: 191 mg

Ingredients:

- 1/4 teaspoon freshly ground black pepper
- 1 tablespoon fresh lemon juice
- 1/4 teaspoon finely grated lemon zest
- 1/2 cup no-salt-added vegetable stock (or broth)
- 1 pound Brussels sprouts (trimmed and quartered)
- 1/4 teaspoon salt (divided)
- 3 shallots (thinly sliced)
- 3 teaspoons extra-virgin olive oil (divided)

Directions:

1. Heat 2 tablespoons of oil in a pan over medium flame. Add shallots and cook for 6 minutes while stirring often. Add 1/8 teaspoon of salt. Stir and transfer to a bowl.

2. Heat the rest of the oil in the same pan over medium flame. Sauté the Brussels sprouts for 4 minutes. Add the stock and simmer for 6 minutes. Put the shallots back to the pan. Stir

in pepper, salt, 1/8 teaspoon of salt, and lemon zest and juice.

Baked Beans

Serves: 12

Calories per serving: 152

Sodium per serving: 215 mg

Ingredients:

- 3 strips thick-cut bacon (chopped)
- 1 1/2 tablespoons dry mustard
- 1/2 cup light molasses
- 1 yellow onion (chopped)
- 3/4 teaspoon salt (divided)
- 2 bay leaves
- 4 cups water
- 2 cups dried small white beans (picked over, rinsed, soaked overnight, and drained)

Directions:

1. Put half a teaspoon of salt, bay leaves, water, and beans in a Dutch oven over high flame. Mix well. Bring to a boil. Turn heat to low and partially cover the pan. Simmer for 75 minutes or until the beans are soft. Discard the bay leaf and turn off the heat.

2. Add 1/4 teaspoon of salt, bacon, mustard, molasses, and onion to the beans. Cover the pan and bake in a preheated oven at 350 degrees F for 5 hours. Occasionally check to stir and add hot water if necessary.

Apples and Acorn Squash

Serves: 2

Calories per serving: 204

Sodium per serving: 46 mg

Ingredients:

- 2 teaspoons trans fat-free margarine
- 1 small acorn squash
- 2 tablespoons brown sugar
- 1 Granny Smith apple (peeled, cored, and sliced)

Directions:

1. Put brown sugar and apple in a bowl. Mix well.

2. Use a sharp knife to pierce the squash several times. Cook in the microwave for 3 minutes or until tender. Turn it over and microwave for 2 more minutes. Transfer to a cutting board and divide into 2. Remove the

seeds and scoop the apple mixture in the hollow part. Microwave for 2 minutes.

3. Transfer to a plate and top with margarine before serving.

Creamy Swiss Chard

Serves: 8

Calories per serving: 80

Sodium per serving: 265 mg

Ingredients:

- 1 tablespoon grated Parmesan cheese
- 1/2 teaspoon freshly ground black pepper
- 2 pounds Swiss chard (rinsed, stemmed and cut into strips)
- 1 1/4 cups low-fat plain soy milk
- 3 garlic cloves (minced)
- 1 1/2 tablespoons unbleached all-purpose flour
- 2 tablespoons olive oil

Directions:

1. Heat oil in a pan over medium flame. Add flour and whisk until it turns into a paste. Add garlic and cook for 30 seconds. Stir in soy milk.

Cook until slightly thick. Put the chard and mix until coated. Cover the pan and cook for 2 minutes or until tender. Season with pepper.

2. Top with Parmesan cheese before serving.

Wild Rice and Apples

Serves: 8

Calories per serving: 213

Sodium per serving: 6 mg

Ingredients:

- 2 Granny Smith apples (cored and diced)
- 1 tablespoon sugar
- 1 tablespoon red wine vinegar
- 2 tablespoons olive oil
- 1/2 cup dried cranberries (no sugar added)
- 1 1/2 cups wild rice (rinsed and drained)
- 3 cups water
- 1/4 cup slivered almonds

Directions:

1. Bake almonds in a preheated oven at 325 degrees F for 10 minutes. Transfer to a bowl and leave to cool.

2. Pour 3 cups of water in a saucepan over medium-high flame. Bring to a boil. Add rice, turn heat to low and cover the pan. Simmer for an hour while checking often and adding water as needed. Drain and put the cooked rice back to the pan. Add the cranberries and mix well. Cover the pan to retain heat.

3. Whisk sugar, vinegar, and oil in a bowl until combined.

4. Put diced apples and rice in a bowl. Mix until combined. Add oil and toss to coat. Add toasted almonds before serving.

Wild Rice Stuffing

Serves: 12

Calories per serving: 91

Sodium per serving: 116 mg

Ingredients:

- 1 cup chopped apple (including peel)
- 1 cup sliced mushrooms
- 3/4 cup chopped onion
- 1 tablespoon olive oil
- 2 1/2 cups water
- 3/4 cup uncooked wild rice
- 1/4 cup slivered almonds, toasted

- 1/2 cup reduced-sodium chicken broth
- 1 tablespoon poultry seasoning
- 1/4 teaspoon black pepper
- 1/2 teaspoon salt
- 2 cups diced celery
- 1/4 cup dried cranberries

Directions:

1. Rinse wild rice thoroughly. Put in a pan with water over medium-high flame. Bring to a boil. Turn heat to low, cover the pan and simmer for 30 minutes while constantly stirring.

2. Heat oil in a pan over medium flame. Add celery, cranberries, apple, mushrooms, and onion. Cook until tender while stirring often. Add poultry seasoning, pepper, and salt. Cook for 10 minutes.

3. Combine chicken broth, vegetable and fruit mixture, and rice in a bowl. Bake for 20 minutes or until warmed.

4. Garnish with toasted almonds before serving. You can also use this dish as stuffing for turkey.

Roasted Beets with Thyme

Serves: 4

Calories per serving: 59

Sodium per serving: 179 mg

Ingredients:

- 1/4 teaspoon ground black pepper
- 1/4 teaspoon salt
- 1 teaspoon fresh thyme
- 1 tablespoon olive oil
- 2 medium golden or red beets (rinsed and trimmed)

Directions:

1. Put beets in foil, wrap and bake in a preheated oven at 400 degrees F for 40 minutes. Leave to cool. Peel and cut into chunks.

2. Put the cooked beets in a bowl. Add pepper, salt, thyme, and oil. Mix well. Transfer to a baking sheet and cook in the oven for 10 minutes.

Spiced Green Beans

Serves: 10

Calories per serving: 42

Sodium per serving: 72 mg

Ingredients:

- 1/8 teaspoon garlic powder
- 1/4 teaspoon pepper
- 1/4 teaspoon salt
- 1 1/2 teaspoons mustard
- 1 1/2 teaspoons vinegar
- 4 1/2 teaspoons water
- 4 1/2 teaspoons olive oil or canola oil
- 1/3 cup diced sweet red bell peppers
- 1 1/2 pounds green beans (fresh, frozen or canned)

Directions:

1. Steam red peppers and beans until crisp-tender.

2. Put the rest of the ingredients in a bowl. Whisk until combined.

3. Pour sauce over the veggies and toss until coated.

Tabbouleh Salad

Serves: 8

Calories per serving: 108

Sodium per serving: 28 mg

Ingredients:

- 1 cup chopped parsley
- 1 cup tomatoes (seeded and diced)
- 3/4 cup bulgur (rinsed and drained)
- 1 1/2 cups water
- 1/4 cup lemon juice
- 1/4 cup raisins
- 4 black olives (sliced)
- 1 teaspoon dill weed
- 1/2 cup chopped scallions or green onions
- Freshly ground black pepper to taste
- 2 tablespoons extra-virgin olive oil

Directions:

1. Put water in a pan over medium-high flame. Bring to a boil. Turn off the heat and add the bulgur. Cover the pan and leave for 20 minutes. Transfer bulgur to a bowl. Add the rest of the ingredients. Toss until combined.

2. Cover the bowl and keep in the fridge for 2 hours.

Sweetened Carrots

Serves: 4

Calories per serving: 40

Sodium per serving: 202 mg

Ingredients:

- 1 teaspoon lemon juice
- Sugar substitute to taste
- 4 tablespoons fresh parsley (chopped)
- 1 teaspoon trans-free margarine
- 2 cups shredded carrots
- 1/4 teaspoon salt
- 1/2 cup water

Directions:

1. Boil water in a pan over medium-high flame. Add shredded carrots and salt. Cover the pan and cook for 5 minutes. Transfer carrots to a bowl. Add parsley, lemon juice, sugar substitute, and margarine. Mix until combined.

2. Serve at once.

Spiced Cabbage

Serves: 6

Calories per serving: 148

Sodium per serving: 35 mg

Ingredients:

- 1 teaspoon cumin seed
- 1/4 teaspoon ground cloves
- 1 teaspoon ground cinnamon
- 1 garlic clove (crushed)
- 1 cup pitted prunes (chopped)
- 1 tart apple (cored, peeled, and chopped)
- 2 medium onions (chopped)
- 1 1/2 pounds red cabbage (cored, quartered, and shredded)
- 1/2 cup water
- Ground nutmeg to taste
- 2 tablespoons red wine vinegar
- 1 teaspoon coriander seed

Directions:

1. Put all ingredients in a pot over medium-high flame. Mix well. Cover the pot and cook for an hour while constantly stirring. Add water as needed.

2. Transfer to a bowl and serve.

Shrimp Ceviche with Cucumber

Serves: 8

Calories per serving: 98

Sodium per serving: 167 mg

Ingredients:

- 1 cup diced tomato
- 1/2 cup diced red onion
- 2 teaspoons cumin
- 2 tablespoons olive oil
- 2 limes (zest and juice)
- 2 lemons (zest and juice)
- 1/2 pound raw shrimp (cut in 1/4-inch pieces)
- 1/4 cup chopped cilantro
- 1 cup cucumber (peeled, diced, and seeded)
- 1/4 cup serrano chili pepper (diced and seeded)
- 1 cup black beans (cooked)
- 2 tablespoons minced garlic

Directions:

1. Put shrimp in a pan. Add lime and lemon juice. Reserve the zest. Keep in the fridge for 3 hours.

2. Put the rest of the ingredients in another bowl. Mix well. Add the cold-cooked shrimp. Toss until combined.

3. Serve dish as is or with baked tortilla chips.

Roasted Green Beans with Tomatoes

Serves: 6

Calories per serving: 59

Sodium per serving: 132 mg

Ingredients:

- 1/2 teaspoon pepper
- 1/2 teaspoon salt
- 1 teaspoon onion powder
- 1 teaspoon dried oregano
- 1 teaspoon dried basil
- 2 teaspoons olive oil
- 1 tablespoon minced garlic
- 1 cup cherry tomatoes
- 2 cups green beans (rinsed and trimmed)

Directions:

1. Put oregano, basil, oil, garlic, tomatoes, pepper, salt, onion powder, and trimmed green beans in a bowl. Toss until combined. Arrange

on a lightly greased baking sheet. Roast in a preheated oven at 400 degrees F for 15 minutes while stirring every 5 minutes.

Butternut Squash Fries

Serves: 6

Calories per serving: 62

Sodium per serving: 168 mg

Ingredients:

- 1/2 teaspoon salt
- 1 tablespoon chopped fresh rosemary
- 1 tablespoon chopped fresh thyme
- 1 tablespoon olive oil
- 1 medium butternut squash

Directions:

1. Peel butternut squash and slice into sticks. Transfer to a bowl. Add salt, rosemary, thyme, and oil. Toss until coated. Arrange on a lightly greased baking sheet. Roast in a preheated oven at 425 degrees F for 10 minutes. Shake and continue baking until golden brown. This will take about 5 to 10 minutes.

Ratatouille with Vinaigrette

Serves: 8

Calories per serving: 84

Sodium per serving: 152 mg

Ingredients:

- 2 zucchini (cut into 1/2-inch cubes)
- 7 teaspoons extra-virgin olive oil (divided)
- 1 eggplant (cut into 1/2-inch cubes)
- 1 tablespoon chopped fresh flat-leaf parsley
- 1 tablespoon chopped fresh basil
- 1 tablespoon grated lemon zest
- 1/2 teaspoon freshly ground black pepper
- 1/2 teaspoon salt
- 1/4 cup balsamic vinegar
- 1 shallot (coarsely chopped)
- 1 red bell pepper (roasted and seeded)
- 1 yellow bell pepper (roasted and seeded)
- 2 plum tomatoes (halved lengthwise)

Directions:

1. Put eggplant and a teaspoon of olive oil in a bowl. Toss until coated. Arrange in a greased baking sheet.

2. Put zucchini in the same bowl and add a tablespoon of oil. Toss until combined. Arrange in another greased baking sheet. Add the tomato halves on top. Brush the remaining oil o the surface of the tomatoes.

3. Put the zucchini and tomatoes in the oven's middle rack and the eggplant on the lower rack. Toast for 8 minutes. Leave to cool.

4. Peel and dice the roasted bell peppers.

5. Prepare the vinaigrette. Put pepper, salt, balsamic vinegar, shallot, and roasted tomatoes in a food processor or blender. Process until combined and smooth. Gradually add 5 teaspoons of olive oil as you blend.

6. Put lemon zest, bell peppers, zucchini, and eggplant in a bowl. Mix well. Add the vinaigrette and mix until coated. Add parsley and basil. Cover the bowl and refrigerate before serving.

Roasted Cheesy Cauliflower

Serves: 6

Calories per serving: 84

Sodium per serving: 163 mg

Ingredients:

- 3 cups small cauliflower florets
- 1/4 teaspoon kosher salt
- 1/4 teaspoon paprika
- 1 teaspoon finely chopped fresh basil
- 1 teaspoon fresh lemon zest
- 2 tablespoons olive oil
- 1/4 cup finely grated Parmesan cheese
- 1/2 cup panko bread crumbs

Directions:

1. Put water in a pot over and bring to a boil. Turn off the heat.

2. Mix to combine salt, paprika, basil, lemon zest, oil, cheese, and bread crumbs in a bowl. Mash using your fingers until well-combined.

3. Soak cauliflower in boiling water for 3 minutes. Drain and transfer to a baking dish. Top with the breadcrumb mixture. Bake in a preheated oven at 375 degrees for 15 minutes.

Lentil Ragout

Serves: 6

Calories per serving: 152

Sodium per serving: 179 mg

Ingredients:

- 1/4 teaspoon ground black pepper
- 1 teaspoon kosher salt
- 4 garlic cloves (minced)
- 1 tablespoon chopped fresh thyme
- 1 cup raw red lentils
- 5 cups water
- 6 medium tomatoes (chopped)
- 1 cup chopped onions
- 1 teaspoon olive oil

Directions:

1. Heat oil in a saucepan over medium-high flame. Add onions and cook for 3 minutes. Stir in tomatoes and cook for 3 more minutes. Add lentils and water. Cook for 20 minutes or until most of the water is gone. Stir in pepper, salt, garlic, and thyme.

Country-Style Sausage

Serves: 6

Calories per serving: 109

Sodium per serving: 52 mg

Ingredients:

- 1 teaspoon dry mustard
- 1 teaspoon sugar
- 1/2 pound lean ground turkey breast
- 1/2 pound lean ground pork loin
- 1/2 teaspoon red pepper flakes (optional)
- 1 teaspoon ground black pepper
- 1 teaspoon sage
- 1 teaspoon onion powder

Directions:

1. Put all ingredients in a bowl. Mix well. Use your hands to shape the mixture into 12 patties.

2. Coat skillet with cooking spray over medium flame. Put the patties and cover the skillet. Cook each side for 5 minutes or until browned. Transfer to a plate and serve at once.

Sweet Potatoes with Glaze

Serves: 8

Calories per serving: 150

Sodium per serving: 42 mg

Ingredients:

- 2 pounds sweet potatoes (peeled and sliced into wedges)
- 1 tablespoon olive oil
- 2 tablespoons honey
- Cracked black pepper to taste
- 2 tablespoons brown sugar
- 1/4 cup water

Directions:

1. Prepare the sauce. Whisk olive oil, honey, brown sugar, and water in a bowl until combined.

2. Arrange potatoes on a single layer in a greased baking tray. Top with sauce. Flip the pieces and cover the other side with sauce. Cover the tray and bake in a preheated oven at 375 degrees F for 45 minutes. Turn and cover the potatoes with sauce every 10 minutes. Continue baking without a cover for 15 minutes.

3. Transfer to a plate and top with your preferred herbs and pepper.

Veggie and Chicken Wraps

Serves: 8

Calories per serving: 214

Sodium per serving: 229 mg

Ingredients:

- 1 cup frozen shelled edamame

For the wraps:

- 8 whole wheat tortillas (room temperature)
- 1 cup cooked chicken breast (chopped)
- 1/2 cup sweet red pepper (thinly sliced)
- 1/2 cup shredded carrots
- 1 cup fresh sugar snap peas (chopped)
- 1 cup thinly sliced cucumber
- 2 cups fresh baby spinach

For the dressing:

- 1/8 teaspoon pepper
- 1/4 teaspoon salt
- 1/2 teaspoon ground ginger
- 1 teaspoon sesame oil
- 2 tablespoons olive oil
- 2 tablespoons orange juice

Directions:

1. Cook edamame according to the directions indicated in its package. Drain liquid and rinse with cold water. Drain liquid and set aside.

2. Put all ingredients for the dressing in a bowl. Whisk until combined.

3. Put chicken and the rest of the vegetables in the bowl with the cooked edamame. Add dressing and gently toss until coated. Scoop half a cup of the mixture to each piece of tortilla. Fold and roll up each filled tortilla.

Chicken and Cherry Lettuce Wraps

Serves: 4

Calories per serving: 257

Sodium per serving: 381 mg

Ingredients:

- 8 Boston lettuce leaves
- 1 tablespoon honey
- 2 tablespoons teriyaki sauce (reduced-sodium)
- 2 tablespoons rice vinegar
- 1/3 cup almonds (coarsely chopped)
- 4 green onions (chopped)
- 1 1/4 cups pitted fresh sweet cherries (coarsely chopped)
- 1 1/2 cups shredded carrots
- 2 teaspoons olive oil
- 1/4 teaspoon pepper
- 1/4 teaspoon salt
- 1 teaspoon ground ginger

- 3/4 pound skinless and boneless chicken breasts (cut into 3/4-inch cubes)

Directions:

1. Season meat with pepper, salt, and ginger.

2. Heat oil in a pan over medium-high flame. Cook the seasoned chicken for 5 minutes. Transfer to a bowl. Add almonds, green onions, cherries, and carrots. Gently toss.

3. Put honey, teriyaki sauce, and vinegar in a bowl. Mix well and add to the meat mixture. Spoon filling in each lettuce leaf. Fold lettuce to secure filling.

Asparagus with Horseradish Dip

Serves: 16

Calories per serving (1 tablespoon of dip and 2 asparagus spears): 63

Sodium per serving: 146 mg

Ingredients:

- 1/2 teaspoon Worcestershire sauce

- 1 tablespoon prepared horseradish
- 1/4 cup grated Parmesan cheese
- 1 cup mayonnaise (reduced-fat)
- 32 fresh asparagus spears (trimmed)

Directions:

1. Steam asparagus until crisp and tender. This will take about 4 minutes. Drain excess moist and place in water with ice. Drain liquid and place asparagus in paper towels. Transfer to a plate.

2. Put the rest of the ingredients in a bowl. Mix well. Drizzle over the cooked asparagus and serve at once.

Spicy Almonds

Serves: 2 1/2 cups

Calories per serving (1/4 cup): 230

Sodium per serving: 293 mg

Ingredients:

- 2 1/2 cups almonds (unblanched)
- 1 egg white (room temperature)

- 1/4 teaspoon cayenne pepper
- 1/2 teaspoon ground coriander
- 1/2 teaspoon ground cumin
- 1/2 teaspoon ground cinnamon
- 1 teaspoon paprika
- 1 1/2 teaspoons kosher salt
- 1 tablespoon sugar

Directions:

1. Put cayenne pepper, coriander, salt, sugar, cumin, cinnamon, and paprika in a bowl. Mix until combined.

2. Put the egg whites in another bowl and whisk until foamy. Add the spice mixture and almonds. Toss until coated.

3. Transfer to a baking pan and even spread in a single layer. Bake in a preheated oven at 325 degrees for half an hour while stirring every 10 minutes. Transfer to a waxed paper and leave to cool.

4. Store leftovers in an airtight container.

Cannellini Bean Hummus

Serves: 10

Calories per serving (2 tablespoons): 78

Sodium per serving: 114 mg

Ingredients:

- 2 tablespoons fresh parsley (minced)
- 1/4 teaspoon red pepper flakes (crushed)
- 1/4 teaspoon salt
- 1 1/2 teaspoons ground cumin
- Assorted fresh veggies
- Pita breads (sliced cut into wedges)
- 3 tablespoons lemon juice
- 1/4 cup tahini
- 1 15-ounce can cannellini beans (rinsed and drained)
- 2 garlic cloves (peeled and minced)

Directions:

1. Put beans, minced garlic, pepper flakes, salt, cumin, lemon juice, and tahini in a food processor. Process until combined and smooth. Transfer to a bowl and add parsley. Stir and place in the fridge until ready to serve.

2. You can serve this along with sliced fresh veggies or pita wedges.

Zucchini with Italian Sausage Stuffing

Serves: 6

Calories per serving (2 zucchini halves): 206

Sodium per serving: 485 mg

Ingredients:

- 3/4 cup shredded part-skim mozzarella cheese
- 1/4 teaspoon pepper
- 2 tablespoons fresh basil (minced)
- 2 tablespoons fresh oregano (minced)
- 1/3 cup minced fresh parsley, add more for toppings
- 1/3 cup grated Parmesan cheese
- 1 cup panko bread crumbs
- 2 medium tomatoes (seeded and chopped)
- 1 pound Italian turkey sausage links (casings removed)
- 6 medium zucchinis (cut in half)

Directions:

1. Scoop out pulp from each zucchini slice. Chop pulp and place in a bowl.

2. Arrange zucchini shells in a heatproof container. Cover and microwave in batches until crisp and tender. This will take about 3 minutes on high setting. Add pepper, herbs,

Parmesan cheese, breadcrumbs, and tomatoes. Turn off the heat.

3. Put zucchini pulp in a pan over medium-high flame. Stir in sausage and cook for 6 minutes while breaking meat into crumbles.

4. Scoop filling to each zucchini shell. Arrange them in a baking pan, cover, and bake in a preheated oven for 20 minutes. Remove the cover and add mozzarella cheese on top. Continue baking for 8 minutes.

5. Top with minced parsley before serving.

Quinoa and Vegetable Dip

Serves: 32

Calories per serving: 65

Sodium per serving: 54 mg

Ingredients:

- 1/4 cup red onion (finely chopped)
- 3/4 cup zucchini (finely chopped)
- 3/4 cup cucumber (peeled, seeded, and chopped)
- 3 plum tomatoes (chopped)
- 1/4 cup fresh cilantro (minced)
- 2 tablespoons, plus 3/4 cup sour cream

- 2 medium ripe avocados (peeled and chopped)
- 5 tablespoons lime juice (divided)
- 2/3 cup quinoa (rinsed)
- Cucumber slices
- Salt and pepper to taste
- 1 2/3 cups water (divided)
- 1/2 teaspoon cayenne pepper
- 1 1/2 teaspoons paprika
- 1 1/2 teaspoons ground cumin
- 2 15-ounce cans black beans (rinsed and drained)

Directions:

1. Put 1/3 cup of water, cayenne, paprika, cumin, and beans in a food processor. Pulse until smooth. Season with salt and pepper.

2. Cook quinoa with 1 1/3 cups of water in a pan over medium-high flame. Turn off the heat and add 2 tablespoons of lime juice. Fluff quinoa with fork.

3. Put the rest of the lime juice, cilantro, 2 tablespoons of sour cream, and avocado in a bowl. Mash the avocado as you mix.

4. Place the bean mixture in a dish. Top with the quinoa mixture. Spread avocado mixture on top and the rest of the sour cream, onion, zucchini, chopped cucumber, and tomatoes.

5. Serve along with cucumber slices.

Chapter 8 – Soup Recipes

Asparagus Soup

Serves: 12

Calories per serving (3/4 cup): 79

Sodium per serving: 401 mg

Ingredients:

- 6 cups chicken broth (reduced-sodium)
- 2/3 cup long-grain brown rice (uncooked)
- 1/4 teaspoon dried thyme
- 1/4 teaspoon pepper
- Salad croutons (optional)
- Reduced-fat sour cream (optional)
- 1/2 teaspoon salt
- 1 medium carrot (sliced)
- 1 medium onion (chopped)
- 2 pounds fresh asparagus (trimmed and chopped)
- 1 tablespoon olive oil
- 1 tablespoon butter

Directions:

1. Heat oil and butter in a stockpot over medium flame. Add the veggies and seasonings and cook for 10 minutes while stirring every now and then. Add broth and rice. Bring to a boil. Turn heat to low and cover the pot. Simmer for 45 minutes while occasionally stirring.

2. Use an immersion blender to puree the soup. You can serve this along with croutons and sour cream.

Notes: You can prepare this soup in advance. Place in a container, cover, and freeze. Partially thaw in the refrigerator overnight. Reheat in a saucepan over medium flame while whisking often.

Beef and Veggie Soup

Serves: 8

Calories per serving: 207

Sodium per serving: 621 mg

Ingredients:

- 4 14.5-ounce cans reduced-sodium beef broth
- 1/2 cup cut green beans (fresh or frozen)
- 1 medium red potato (finely chopped)

- 1 medium zucchini (coarsely chopped)
- 1 1/2 cups shredded cabbage
- 1 14.5-ounce can diced tomatoes (with the liquid)
- 1/4 cup tomato paste
- 2 celery ribs (chopped)
- 1 10-ounce package julienned carrots
- 2 garlic cloves (minced)
- 1 medium onion (chopped)
- 1 1/2 pounds lean ground beef (90 percent lean)
- Grated Parmesan cheese (optional)
- 1/4 teaspoon pepper
- 1/4 teaspoon salt
- 1/2 teaspoon dried oregano
- 1 teaspoon dried basil

Directions:

1. Put beef in a stockpot over medium flame. Add garlic and onion and cook for 8 minutes. Break meat into crumbles as you cook. Drain cooking liquid and return to heat. Add celery and carrots. Cook for 8 minutes. Add tomato paste and stir for a minute.

2. Add broth, seasonings, green beans, potato, zucchini, cabbage, and tomatoes. Bring to a boil. Turn heat to low and cover the pot. Simmer for 45 minutes.

3. Top with cheese before serving.

Green Bean and Tomato Soup

Serves: 9

Calories per serving (1 cup): 58

Sodium per serving: 535 mg

Ingredients:

- 1/4 teaspoon pepper
- 1/2 teaspoon salt
- 1/4 cup fresh basil (minced)
- 3 cups fresh tomatoes (diced)
- 1 garlic clove (minced)
- 1 pound fresh green beans (cut into smaller pieces)
- 6 cups vegetable or chicken broth (reduced-sodium)
- 2 teaspoons butter
- 1 cup chopped carrots
- 1 cup chopped onion

Directions:

1. Melt butter in a pan over medium flame. Add carrots and onion and cook for 5 minutes. Add garlic, beans, and broth. Bring to a boil. Turn heat to low and cover the pan. Simmer for 20 minutes. Add salt, pepper, basil, and tomatoes. Cover the pan and simmer for 5 more minutes.

Beef Stew with Veggies

Serves: 6

Calories per serving: 244

Sodium per serving: 185 mg

Ingredients:

- 3 tablespoons all-purpose flour
- 4 large white or red-skinned potatoes (peeled and chunked)
- 18 small boing onions (cut into 2 crosswise)
- 3 portobello mushrooms (cleaned with a brush, chunked)
- 1/3 cup fresh flat-leaf parsley (minced)
- 2 fresh thyme sprigs
- 3/4 teaspoon ground black pepper (divided)
- 1 bay leaf

- 3 cups salt-free vegetable stock
- 1/2 cup red wine (optional)
- 4 large carrots (peeled and chunked)
- 1 pound boneless lean beef stew meat (visible fat trimmed, cubed)
- 2 tablespoons canola or olive oil
- 1/2 fennel bulb (trimmed and thinly sliced)
- 3 large shallots (chopped)

Directions:

1. Dredge meat in flour. Heat oil in a pan over medium flame. Cook beef until all sides are browned. Transfer to a plate and set aside.

2. Reduce the stove's heat to medium. Add shallots and fennel to the pan. Sauté for 8 minutes or until lightly golden. Stir in bay leaf, thyme sprigs, and 1/4 teaspoon of pepper. Cook for a minute. Add the cooked beef, wine, and vegetable stock. Bring to a boil. Cover the pan and turn heat to low. Simmer for 45 minutes or until the meat is tender.

3. Stir in mushroom, onions, potatoes, and carrots. Simmer for 30 minutes. Remove bay leaf and thyme sprigs. Add the rest of the pepper and parsley.

4. Transfer to a bowl and serve at once.

Cream of Wild Rice Hot Dish

Serves: 4

Calories per serving: 236

Sodium per serving: 180 mg

Ingredients:

- 2 cloves garlic, minced
- 1 cup diced celery
- 1 cup diced carrot
- 1 1/2 cups diced yellow onion
- 1/2 tablespoon canola oil
- 1 teaspoon fennel seeds, crushed
- 2 cups low-sodium vegetable stock
- 1 tablespoon minced parsley
- 1 1/2 cups chopped kale
- 1/2 cup wild rice, cooked
- 1 teaspoon ground black pepper
- 2 cups 1 percent milk
- 1 cup unsalted prepared white beans (or about 1/2 of a 15.5 ounce can of white beans, rinsed and drained)

Directions:

1. Heat oil in a soup pot over medium flame. Add garlic, celery, carrot, and onion. Cook until

browned while constantly stirring. Add spices, stock, parsley, and kale. Stir and bring to a boil.

2. Put milk and beans in a food processor. Process until pureed. Transfer to a pot with soup. Add rice and simmer for half an hour.

Tasty Carrot Soup

Serves: 6

Calories per serving: 140

Sodium per serving: 164 mg

Ingredients:

- 2 cups water
- 1 1/2 tablespoons sugar
- 10 carrots (peeled and sliced)
- 2 tablespoons fresh parsley (chopped)
- 4 cups fat-free milk
- 1/4 teaspoon ground nutmeg
- 1/4 teaspoon ground black pepper
- 3 tablespoons all-purpose flour

Directions:

1. Put water, sugar, and carrots in a saucepan over medium flame. Cover the pan and simmer for 20 minutes. Sift the carrots while reserving some of the cooking liquid.

2. Prepare the white sauce. Put milk, nutmeg, pepper, and flour in another saucepan over medium-high flame. Whisk mixture until thick.

3. Transfer white sauce to a food processor. Add the cooked carrots and process until pureed. Gradually add the reserved cooking liquid to get your preferred consistency. Scoop into serving bowls and top with parsley.

Curried Carrot Soup

Serves: 6

Calories per serving: 104

Sodium per serving: 116 mg

Ingredients:

- 1 tablespoon, plus 1 teaspoon fresh ginger (peeled and chopped)
- 1 pound carrots (peeled and cut small pieces)
- 1/2 yellow onion (chopped)
- 1 teaspoon mustard seed
- 1 tablespoon olive oil
- 1/4 cup chopped fresh cilantro, plus leaves for garnish
- 5 cups low-sodium chicken stock (or broth or vegetable stock)

- 2 teaspoons curry powder
- 1/2 jalapeno (seeded)
- 3 tablespoons low-fat sour cream
- Grated zest of 1 lime
- 1/2 teaspoon salt (optional)
- 2 tablespoons fresh lime juice

Directions:

1. Heat oil in a pan over medium flame. Put the mustard seed and stir for a minute. Stir in onion and cook for 4 minutes. Add curry powder, jalapeno, ginger, and carrots. Cook for 3 minutes. Add 3 cups of stock and turn the heat to high. Leave until it boils. Turn heat to medium-low and simmer for 6 minutes.

2. Use an immersion blender to puree the soup or process it in a blender or food processor in batches.

3. Heat soup in a pot over medium flame. Add 2 cups of stock. Turn off the flame and add lime juice and chopped cilantro.

4. Put cilantro leaves, lemon zest or a drizzle of yogurt on top before serving.

Yummy Asparagus Soup

Serves: 6

Calories per serving: 140

Sodium per serving: 76 mg

Ingredients:

- 1/2 cup chopped onion
- 1/2 pound fresh asparagus (chopped)
- 2 cups potatoes (peeled and diced)
- 2 tablespoons butter
- 4 cups water
- 2 celery stalks (chopped)
- Cracked black pepper to taste
- Lemon zest to taste
- 1 1/2 cups fat-free milk
- 1/2 cup whole-wheat flour

Directions:

1. Pour water in a pot over high flame. Add celery, onions, asparagus, and potatoes. Bring to a boil. Turn heat to low and cover the pot. Simmer for 15 minutes or until tender. Add butter and stir until incorporated.

2. Mix to combine milk and flour in a bowl. Gradually add to the soup in the pot as you stir. Turn heat to medium-high. Stir soup until

thick. Turn off the heat and season with cracked black pepper and lemon zest.

Turkey Soup

Serves: 10

Calories per serving: 178

Sodium per serving: 131 mg

Ingredients:

For the broth:

- 3 large onions (chop the 3 and cut the other into quarters)
- 8 cups low-sodium chicken broth
- 4 cups water
- 1 turkey carcass

For the soup:

- 1/4 teaspoon dried thyme
- 1/4 cup chopped fresh parsley
- 4 carrots (peeled and sliced into thin strips)
- 1 cup chopped celery
- 1 cup diced rutabaga (peeled)
- 1 onion (chopped)

- 1/2 pound leftover light turkey meat (chunked)
- 1 16-ounce can white beans (rinsed and drained)
- 1 14-ounces can unsalted tomatoes
- 1/4 cup uncooked pearl barley
- 1/2 teaspoon ground black pepper
- 1 bay leaf

Directions:

1. Put water, onion, broth, and turkey carcass in a pot over high flame. Bring to a boil. Turn heat to low and cover the pot. Simmer for an hour.

2. Strain soup to remove onion and carcass. Transfer soup to a bowl. Skim off visible fat at the surface, cover the bowl and keep in the fridge overnight.

3. Heat broth mixture in a pot over low flame. Add ingredients for the soup and cover the pot. Simmer for an hour and serve at once.

Chickpea and Tomato Soup

Serves: 6

Calories per serving: 125

Sodium per serving: 156 mg

Ingredients:

- 1/4 teaspoon hot pepper sauce
- 1/4 cup fresh cilantro or parsley (chopped)
- 1/4 cup red onion (chopped)
- 1/2 cup cucumber (seeded and chopped)
- 1 cup cherry tomatoes (quartered)
- 6 cups unsalted vegetable juice
- 1 15-ounce can chickpeas (rinsed and drained)
- 6 lime wedges
- 1/4 cup lime juice
- 3 garlic cloves (minced)

Directions:

1. Put lime juice, garlic, hot pepper sauce, cilantro, onion, cucumber, tomatoes, vegetable juice, and chickpeas in a bowl. Mix until combined. Cover the bowl and chill in the fridge for at least an hour.

2. Scoop in chilled individuals bowls and top with lime wedge before serving.

Roasted Corn Soup

Serves: 12

Calories per serving: 119

Sodium per serving: 184 mg

Ingredients:

- 2 cups carrots (chopped)
- 3 cups onion (chopped)
- 1 1/2 tablespoons olive oil
- 4 cups corn kernels
- 1/4 cup all-purpose flour
- 2 teaspoons chopped garlic
- 2 cups chopped celery
- 1 tablespoon chopped parsley
- 1/8 teaspoon white pepper
- 1 teaspoon salt
- 1 1/2 cups half-and-half
- 2 jalapeno peppers (minced)
- 6 cups vegetable stock
- 1 teaspoon cumin

Directions:

1. Roast corn kernels in a preheated oven at 500 degrees F for 8 minutes or until they start to caramelize.

2. Heat oil in a pot over medium-high flame. Add garlic, celery, carrots, and onion. Cook for 5 minutes while constantly stirring. Turn heat to low and add cumin, flour, and corn. Stir for a couple of minutes. Add the jalapenos and vegetable stock. Leave to simmer for half an hour. Add parsley, pepper, salt, and half-and-half.

Basic Vegetable Stock

Serves: 6

Calories per serving: 22

Sodium per serving: 94 mg

Ingredients:

- 3 large carrots (sliced into 1-inch pieces)
- 1 large yellow onion (sliced into 1-inch pieces)
- 14 fresh white mushrooms (brushed clean and coarsely chopped)
- 3 teaspoons olive oil
- 6 fresh flat-leaf parsley sprigs
- 8 cups water
- 6 garlic cloves (halved)
- 2 celery stalks with leaves (sliced into 1-inch pieces)
- 1/8 teaspoon salt
- 1 bay leaf
- 4 fresh thyme sprigs

Directions:

1. Heat 2 teaspoons of oil in a pot over medium-high flame. Add mushrooms and cook for 5 minutes. Push to one side and add the rest of the oil, garlic, celery, carrots, and onion. Turn heat to high and cook veggies for 10 minutes while stirring often. Add water, salt, bay leaf, thyme, and parsley. Bring to a boil. Turn heat to low and simmer for half an hour. Remove from the stove and allow to cool.

2. Strain the stock and use as desired. Put the rest in an airtight container. It will last up to 3 days in the fridge and up to 3 months in the freezer.

Apple and Tomato Soup

Serves: 8

Calories per serving: 205

Sodium per serving: 89 mg

Ingredients:

- 1 tablespoon curry powder
- 1 teaspoon minced garlic
- 1 cup celery (finely chopped)
- 1 1/2 cups onion (finely chopped)
- 2 tablespoons olive oil
- Ground black pepper to taste

- 1/2 teaspoon thyme
- 1 bay leaf
- 3 cups no-salt-added canned tomatoes (drained)
- 1 1/2 cups apple cubes
- 1 cup fat-free milk
- 6 cups low-sodium vegetable broth (or chicken broth)
- 1 cup long-grain brown rice

Directions:

1. Heat oil in a pot over medium flame. Add garlic, celery, and onion and cook for 4 minutes or until tender. Stir in curry powder and cook for a minute. Add rice, black pepper, thyme, bay leaf, and tomatoes. Bring to a boil while stirring often. Add broth and bring to a boil. Turn heat to low and simmer for half an hour. Discard the bay leaf.

2. Transfer soup to a blender or food processor. Process until pureed and smooth. Put back to the pot and add apple cubes and milk. Heat for a couple of minutes.

Pumpkin Soup

Serves: 4

Calories per serving: 77

Sodium per serving: 57 mg

Ingredients:

- 1/4 teaspoon ground nutmeg
- 1/2 teaspoon ground cinnamon
- 2 cups unsalted vegetable broth
- 1 15-ounce can pumpkin puree
- 1 small onion (chopped)
- 3/4 cup water (divided)
- 1 green onion top (chopped)
- 1/8 teaspoon black pepper
- 1 cup fat-free milk

Directions:

1. Put onion and 1/4 cup of water in a pan over medium flame. Cook for 3 minutes or until tender. Add the rest of the water, nutmeg, cinnamon, broth, and pumpkin. Bring to a boil. Turn heat to low and simmer for 5 minutes. Add milk. Turn off heat before it boils.

2. Top with green onion tops and black pepper before serving.

Barley and Mushroom Soup

Serves: 9

Calories per serving: 121

Sodium per serving: 112 mg

Ingredients:

- 3/4 cup chopped carrots
- 1 cup sliced mushrooms
- 1 1/2 cups chopped onions
- 1 tablespoon canola oil
- 1/2 teaspoon chopped garlic
- 1/8 teaspoon black pepper
- 1 teaspoon dried thyme
- 1/4 cup thinly sliced green onions
- 1/2 small potato (chopped)
- 3 ounces dry sherry
- 3/4 cup pearl barley
- 8 cups vegetable stock

Directions:

1. Heat oil in a pot over medium-high flame. Add garlic, pepper, thyme, carrots, mushrooms, and onions. Cook for 5 minutes while stirring often. Add barley and vegetable stock. Bring to a boil. Turn heat to low and simmer for 20 minutes. Add potato and sherry. Simmer for 15 minutes.

2. Top with green onion slices before serving.

Summer Vegetable Hot Dish

Serves: 8

Calories per serving: 62

Sodium per serving: 156 mg

Ingredients:

- 3 garlic cloves (chopped)
- 1 yellow onion (chopped)
- 1 tablespoon olive oil
- 1 teaspoon ground cumin
- 1 tablespoon chopped fresh oregano
- 4 plum tomatoes (peeled, seeded, and diced)
- 1 zucchini (halved and thinly sliced)
- 1 yellow bell pepper (seeded and diced)
- 1 carrot (peeled, halved, and thinly sliced)
- 1 bay leaf
- 4 cups no salt added vegetable stock (or broth)
- 1/4 teaspoon freshly ground black pepper
- 1/4 teaspoon salt
- 2 tablespoons chopped fresh cilantro
- 1 tablespoon grated lemon zest

Directions:

1. Heat oil in a pot over medium flame. Add onion and cook for 4 minutes or until soft. Add garlic and cook for 30 seconds. Stir in tomatoes, cumin, and oregano. Cook for 4 minutes while stirring often. Add leaf bay and stock. Bring to a boil.

2. Turn heat to low and simmer for 10 minutes. Add bell pepper and carrot. Simmer for 2 minutes. Add zucchini and simmer for 3 more minutes. Season with salt and pepper. Stir in cilantro and lemon zest. Remove bay leaf and turn off the flame.

Fennel and Potato Soup

Serves: 8

Calories per serving: 149

Sodium per serving: 104 mg

Ingredients:

- 2 large russet potatoes (peeled and sliced)
- 1 cup chopped red onion
- 1 large fennel bulb (chopped)
- 1 teaspoon olive oil
- 2 teaspoons fennel seeds (toasted)
- 2 teaspoons lemon juice

- 1 cup fat-free milk
- 3 cups reduced-sodium chicken broth

Directions:

1. Heat oil in a pot over medium flame. Add onion and fennel and cook for 5 minutes. Add broth, lemon juice, milk, and potatoes. Turn heat to low and cover the pot. Simmer for 15 minutes.

2. Puree the soup in batches using a food processor or blender. Put back to the pot and cook until heated through.

3. Top with toasted fennel seeds before serving.

Minestrone Soup

Serves: 4

Calories per serving: 213

Sodium per serving: 400 mg

Ingredients:

- 2 tablespoons fresh basil (chopped)
- 1 small zucchini (diced)
- 1/2 cup uncooked whole-grain small shell pasta

- 1 16-ounce can chickpeas or red kidney beans (drained and rinsed)
- 1/2 cup chopped spinach
- 2 large tomatoes (seeded and chopped)
- 4 cups fat-free unsalted chicken broth
- 1 garlic clove (minced)
- 1 carrot (diced)
- 1/3 cup chopped celery
- 1/2 cup chopped onion
- 1 tablespoon olive oil

Directions:

1. Heat oil in a saucepan over medium flame. Add carrots, celery, and onion. Cook for 5 minutes. Stir in garlic and cook for a minute. Add pasta, beans, spinach, and tomatoes. Turn heat to high and bring to a boil. Turn heat to low and simmer for 10 minutes. Add the zucchini, cover the pot and simmer for 5 more minutes. Turn off the heat and add basil.

2. Serve soup at once.

White Bean Stew

Serves: 6

Calories per serving: 307

Sodium per serving: 334 mg

Ingredients:

For the croutons:

- 1 slice whole-grain bread (cubed)
- 2 garlic cloves (quartered)
- 1 tablespoon extra-virgin olive oil

For the soup:

- 1 bay leaf
- 6 cups water
- 2 cups dried cannellini beans (picked over, rinsed, soaked overnight, and drained)
- 1 1/2 cups vegetable stock (or broth)
- 6 sprigs, plus 1 tablespoon chopped fresh rosemary
- 1/4 teaspoon freshly ground black pepper
- 6 cloves garlic (chopped)
- 3 carrots (peeled and coarsely chopped)
- 1 cup yellow onion (coarsely chopped)
- 2 tablespoons olive oil
- 1/2 teaspoon salt (divided)

Directions:

1. Prepare the croutons. Heat oil in a pan over medium flame. Add garlic and cook for a minute. Turn off the heat and leave garlic in the

pan for 10 minutes to infuse its flavor in the oil. Discard garlic and turn on the heat to medium. Stir in bread cubes. Cook for 5 minutes while stirring often. Transfer to a bowl.

2. Prepare the soup. Put water, bay leaf, 1/4 teaspoon of salt, and white beans in a pot over medium-high flame. Bring to a boil. Turn heat to low and partially cover the pot. Simmer for an hour or longer. Check when the beans are tender. Discard bay leaf and drain the beans while reserving half a cup of the liquid. Transfer beans to a bowl.

3. Put half a cup of the cooked beans and the reserved cooking liquid in a bowl. Mash using a fork and add to the cooked beans.

4. Put the pot back in the stove and heat oil over medium-high flame. Add carrots and onion and cook for 7 minutes. Stir in garlic and cook for a minute. Add the stock, bean mixture, chopped rosemary, pepper, and the rest of the salt. Bring to a boil. Turn heat to low and simmer for 5 minutes.

5. Scoop stew into bowls and add rosemary sprigs and croutons on top.

Vegetarian-Friendly Chili Soup

Serves: 8

Calories per serving: 161

Sodium per serving: 116 mg

Ingredients:

- 2 garlic cloves (minced)
- 1 cup diced celery
- 2 cups diced onion
- 2 quarts crushed tomatoes
- 2 Fresno peppers (diced)
- 2 tablespoons water
- 1 cup diced bell pepper
- 1 tablespoon dried oregano
- 1 tablespoon balsamic vinegar
- 1 tablespoon ground black pepper
- 1 tablespoon chipotle pepper (or smoked paprika)
- 2 tablespoons ground cumin
- 2 cups cooked pinto beans (rinsed)

Directions:

1. Heat 2 tablespoons of water in a pot over low flame. Add garlic, bell pepper, celery, and onion. Cook for 10 minutes while stirring often. Stir in the rest of the ingredients. Cover the pot and simmer for 2 hours while occasionally stirring. Add a bit of water if it becomes too thick.

White Chicken Soup with Chili

Serves: 8

Calories per serving: 212

Sodium per serving: 241 mg

Ingredients:

- 1 14.5-ounce can low-sodium diced tomatoes
- 2 15-ounce cans low-sodium white beans (drained)
- 1 10-ounce can white chunk chicken
- 2 garlic cloves (minced)
- 1 medium red pepper (chopped)
- 1/2 medium green pepper (chopped)
- 1 medium onion (chopped)
- 4 cups low-sodium chicken broth
- 1 teaspoon dried oregano
- 1 teaspoon ground cumin
- 2 teaspoons chili powder
- 3 tablespoons chopped fresh cilantro
- 8 tablespoons reduced-fat Monterey Jack cheese (shredded)
- Cayenne pepper to taste

Directions:

1. Put broth, tomatoes, beans, and chicken in a pot over medium flame. Cover and simmer until the meat is cooked.

2. Lightly coat pan with cooking spray and turn heat to medium high. Put garlic, peppers, and onion. Cook for 5 minutes. Turn off the heat and transfer mixture to the soup pot.

3. Stir in cayenne pepper, oregano, cumin, and chili powder to the simmering soup. Simmer for 10 minutes.

4. Top with cilantro and a tablespoon of cheese for each serving.

Quibebe Soup

Serves: 8

Calories per serving: 106

Sodium per serving: 280 mg

Ingredients:

- 1 1/2 garlic cloves (diced)
- 2 Fresno chili peppers (chopped)
- 1 1/2 cups tomatoes (diced)
- 2 cups chopped onions
- 1 tablespoon olive oil

- 2 1/2 tablespoons chopped fresh parsley
- 1/2 teaspoon sugar
- 3/4 teaspoon ground black pepper
- 3/4 teaspoon salt
- 1 butternut squash (cubed)
- 8 cups low-sodium vegetable stock

Directions

1. Heat oil in a pot over medium flame. Add garlic, chili peppers, tomatoes, and onions. Cook for 15 minutes while stirring often. Add squash and vegetable stock. Bring to a boil. Turn heat to low and simmer for 15 minutes or until the squash is tender.

2. Puree soup in a food processor or blender in batches. Put back in the pot. Add sugar, pepper, and salt. Scoop into bowls and top with parsley before serving.

Chicken Stock

Serves: 12

Calories per serving: 16

Sodium per serving: 12 mg

Ingredients:

- 1/4 teaspoon peppercorns
- 1 large yellow onion (chunked)

- 2 celery stalks (sliced into 2-inch pieces)
- 3 carrots (sliced into 2-inch pieces)
- 3 pounds bones from cooked chicken (trim excess fat)
- 4 quarts cold water
- 5 fresh flat-leaf parsley sprigs

Directions

1. Use cold water in rinsing chicken bones. Put in a pan and roast in a preheated oven at 450 degrees F for 20 minutes. Flip the bones and add onion, celery, and carrots. Continue roasting for 20 more minutes.

2. Put the roasted bones and veggies and cold water in a pot over medium-high flame. Put a bit of water in the roasting pan and scrape the sides to deglaze. Transfer liquid to the pot. Add parsley and peppercorns. Bring to a boil. Turn heat to low and simmer for an hour and 30 minutes while partially covered. Scoop out the foam that rises on top as needed. Turn off the heat and leave until slightly cool.

3. Strain the stock. Remove all solids ad bones. Leave at room temperature for an hour to cool. Transfer to a bowl, cover and leave in the fridge overnight.

4. Remove and discard fat at the surface of the broth. Use at once. You can keep the leftovers by storing them in a covered container. It will

last up to 2 days in the fridge and up to 3 months in the freezer.

Cheesy Tomato Soup

Serves: 2

Calories per serving: 178

Sodium per serving: 220

Ingredients:

- 1 tablespoon freshly grated Parmesan cheese
- 2 tablespoons croutons
- 1 tablespoon chopped fresh basil or cilantro
- 1 medium tomato (chopped)
- 1 10.5-ounce can fat-free milk
- 1 1.5-ounce can condensed low-fat, low-sodium tomato soup

Directions:

1. Put milk and soup in a saucepan over medium flame. Whisk for 10 minutes or until smooth. Add herbs and chopped tomato. Cook for 5 minutes while occasionally stirring.

2. Top each serving with 1 1/2 teaspoons of Parmesan cheese and a tablespoon of croutons.

Mushroom and Wild Rice Soup

Serves: 4

Calories per serving: 170

Sodium per serving: 120 mg

Ingredients:

- 1 1/2 cups fresh white mushrooms (sliced)
- 1/4 cup chopped carrots
- 1/4 cup chopped celery
- 1/2 white onion (chopped)
- 1 tablespoon olive oil
- 2 1/2 cups fat-free, low-sodium chicken broth
- 1/2 cup white wine
- Black pepper to taste
- 2 tablespoons flour
- 1 cup fat-free half-and-half
- 1 cup cooked wild rice
- 1/4 teaspoon dried thyme

Directions

1. Heat oil in a pot over medium flame. Add carrots, celery, and onion. Cook for 5 minutes or until tender. Add chicken broth, white wine, and mushrooms. Cover the pot and cook until heated through.

2. Put pepper, thyme, flour, and half-and-half in a bowl. Mix until combined. Add mixture to the cooked rice. Mix well. Transfer to the pot with veggies. Cook until thick and bubbly.

3. Serve while warm.

Bean and Veggie Soup

Serves: 8

Calories per serving: 287

Sodium per serving: 258 mg

Ingredients:

- 1 cup red lentils
- 4 cups low-sodium vegetable stock
- 3 garlic cloves (minced)
- 2 large onions (chopped)
- 3 large carrots (peeled and sliced)
- 3 cups butternut squash (peeled, seeded, and cubed)
- 1 teaspoon turmeric
- 2 teaspoons ground cumin

- 2 tablespoons fresh ginger (peeled and minced)
- 2 tablespoons no-added-salt tomato paste
- 1/2 cup chopped fresh cilantro
- 1/2 cup chopped roasted unsalted peanuts
- 1 16-ounce can garbanzo beans (drained and rinsed)
- 1/4 cup lemon juice
- 1 teaspoon freshly ground pepper
- 1/4 teaspoon saffron

Directions:

1. Put garlic, onions, carrots, and squash in a Dutch oven over medium flame. Stir until onions begin to turn brown. Add the stock, seasonings, tomato paste, and lentils. Scrape the sides and bottom of the pan as you stir. Turn heat to low and cover the pan. Cook for an hour or until the squash and lentils are soft. Stir the dish every now and then. Add garbanzo beans and lemon juice and turn off the heat.

2. Top with cilantro and peanuts before serving.

Turkey Soup with Beans

Serves: 6

Calories per serving: 242

Sodium per serving: 204 mg

Ingredients:

- 3 low-sodium chicken bouillon cubes
- 1 14.5-ounce can unsalted diced tomatoes
- 1/4 cup ketchup
- 1 clove garlic (minced)
- 2 celery stalks (chopped)
- 2 medium onions (chopped)
- 1 pound ground turkey breast
- 1 15-ounce can unsalted cannellini beans (rinsed and drained)
- 2 cups shredded cabbage
- 1/4 teaspoon ground black pepper
- 1 1/2 teaspoons dried basil
- 7 cups water

Directions

1. Put a bit of water in a saucepan over medium-high flame. Add garlic, celery, onion, and turkey. Stir until the turkey is cooked. Add beans, cabbage, pepper, basil, tomatoes, ketchup, water, and bouillon. Bring to a boil. Turn heat to low and cover the pan. Simmer for half an hour.

Roasted Squash Soup

Serves: 4

Calories per serving: 213

Sodium per serving: 139 mg

Ingredients:

- 1 cup diced celery
- 2 teaspoons canola oil (divided)
- 1 small butternut squash (cut into 1/2-inch pieces)
- 2 garlic cloves (minced)
- 1 1/2 cups spinach
- 1 1/2 cups yellow onion (diced)
- 1 teaspoon black pepper
- 1/2 teaspoon nutmeg
- 1 teaspoon sage
- 4 cups unsalted vegetable stock
- 1 cup diced carrot

Directions

1. Put a teaspoon of oil and squash in a roasting pan. Toss until coated. Roast in a preheated oven at 400 degrees F for 40 minutes.

2. Heat the rest of the oil in a pot over medium flame. Add carrot, garlic, spinach, onion, and celery. Sauté for 5 minutes. Add pepper,

nutmeg, sage, stock, and the roasted squash. Simmer for 5 minutes.

3. Puree soup in batches using a food processor or blender. Put the soup back to the pot and simmer for a couple of minutes.

Apple and Potato Soup with Brie

Serves: 8

Calories per serving: 217

Sodium per serving: 220 mg

Ingredients:

- 2 cups low-sodium chicken broth
- 4 large apples (cored, peeled, and quartered)
- 1 large apple for garnish (cored and thinly sliced)
- 1/4 cup sliced leek (white part only)
- 1 cup chopped yellow onion
- 4 ounces Brie (cubed)
- 6 small potatoes (peeled and sliced)
- 3 cups fat-free evaporated milk
- 1/4 teaspoon dried thyme
- 1 bay leaf

Directions

1. Lightly coat pot with a cooking spray and heat over medium flame. Add apples, leeks, and onion. Sauté for 7 minutes while stirring often. Add thyme, bay leaf, and broth. Bring to a boil. Turn heat to low and simmer for 15 minutes. Discard bay leaf and turn off the heat.

2. Put evaporated milk in a saucepan over medium flame. Add the potatoes and cook for 20 minutes or until tender. Constantly whisk the mixture while cooking. Turn off the heat and transfer mixture to the soup pot. Mix well.

3. Puree soup in batches using a blender or food processor while gradually adding pieces of Brie. Put back to the pot and simmer until heated through.

Veggie and Turkey Barley Soup

Serves: 6

Calories per serving: 208

Sodium per serving: 662 mg

Ingredients:

- 1/2 teaspoon pepper
- 2 cups fresh baby spinach
- 2 cups cooked turkey breast (cubed)
- 6 cups chicken broth (reduced-sodium)
- 2/3 cup barley (quick-cooking)

- 1 medium onion (chopped)
- 5 medium carrots (chopped)
- 1 tablespoon canola oil

Directions:

1. Heat oil in a pan over medium-high flame. Add onion and carrots and cook for 5 minutes. Add broth and barley. Bring to a boil. Turn heat to low and cover the pan. Simmer for 15 minutes. Add pepper, spinach, and turkey. Cook until heated through.

Conclusion

I'd like to thank you and congratulate you for transiting my lines from start to finish.

I hope this book was able to help you to understand what the DASH eating plan is all about.

The next step is to stock up on the right ingredients and try the recipes in this book. To gain the maximum benefits from the diet, team it up with a regular exercise routine and a healthy lifestyle.

I wish you the best of luck!